INTRODUCTION

Mesothelioma is a type of cancer that primarily affects the lining of the lungs, and it is often linked to asbestos exposure. Maintaining a healthy and well-balanced diet is essential for overall well-being and can support the body during cancer treatment.

In general, a balanced diet for someone with cancer may include:

1. Adequate Protein: Protein is essential for repairing tissues and maintaining muscle mass, which can be vital during cancer treatment.

2. Healthy Fats: Include sources of healthy fats, such as avocados, nuts, seeds, and olive oil.

3. Fruits and Vegetables: Various colorful fruits and vegetables can provide essential vitamins, minerals, and antioxidants.

4. Whole Grains: Choose whole grains like brown rice, quinoa, and whole wheat for added fiber and nutrients.

5. Hydration: Staying hydrated is essential, especially during cancer treatment. Water, herbal teas, and clear broths can contribute to fluid intake.

6. Small, Frequent Meals: Eating smaller, more frequent meals may be more leisurely for individuals experiencing side effects of treatment, such as nausea or loss of appetite.

As we navigate the complex terrain of mesothelioma and its dietary implications, it becomes evident that empowering individuals with knowledge about the mesothelioma diet is an integral part of a holistic strategy to enhance their resilience, promote healing, and ultimately improve their quality of life in the face of this formidable disease.

CHAPTER ONE

Definition of Mesothelioma

Mesothelioma is a rare and aggressive form of cancer that develops in the mesothelium, a protective membrane lining various internal organs of the body. The mesothelium is composed of two layers: one that surrounds the organ and another that forms a sac-like structure around it. The most common type of mesothelioma occurs in the pleura, the mesothelial tissue surrounding the lungs, but it can also affect the peritoneum (lining of the abdominal cavity), pericardium (sac around the heart), and tunica vaginalis (lining around the testicles).

TYPES OF MESOTHELIOMA

Mesothelioma is a heterogeneous cancer that manifests in various parts of the body, with the most common types being pleural mesothelioma, peritoneal mesothelioma, and pericardial mesothelioma. Each type originates in the mesothelial cells lining specific organs, resulting in distinct sets of symptoms and challenges.

1. Pleural Mesothelioma:

• Location: Pleural mesothelioma is the most prevalent form, affecting the mesothelial lining surrounding the lungs (pleura).

• Symptoms: Common symptoms include chest pain, persistent cough, difficulty breathing, and the accumulation of fluid in the pleural cavity (pleural effusion).

• Causes: Primarily caused by inhalation of asbestos fibers, which become lodged in the pleura, leading to inflammation and cancer development.

• Diagnosis: Diagnosing pleural mesothelioma involves imaging studies, such as CT scans and MRIs, along with biopsy procedures to confirm the presence of malignant cells.

2. Peritoneal Mesothelioma:

• Location: Peritoneal mesothelioma develops in the mesothelial lining of the abdominal cavity (peritoneum).

• Symptoms: Abdominal pain, swelling, changes in bowel habits, and weight loss are common indicators. Peritoneal mesothelioma can also lead to the accumulation of fluid in the abdominal cavity (ascites).

• Causes: Asbestos fibers can reach the peritoneum through ingestion or migration from the pleura. However, the exact mechanism still needs to be fully understood.

• Diagnosis: Diagnosis involves imaging studies and biopsy procedures, often performed during surgery. The presence of specific biomarkers may aid in confirmation.

3. Pericardial Mesothelioma:

• Location: Pericardial mesothelioma is the rarest form, affecting the mesothelial lining around the heart (pericardium).

• Symptoms: Symptoms may include chest pain, irregular heartbeat, difficulty breathing, and fatigue. Due to its location, pericardial mesothelioma can have significant effects on cardiac function.

• Causes: Asbestos exposure is the primary risk factor, similar to other types. However, the rarity of this form limits the available data.

• Diagnosis: Diagnosis involves imaging studies and biopsy procedures, often challenging due to the delicate nature of the pericardium. Advanced imaging techniques may be necessary for accurate assessment.

CAUSES AND RISK FACTORS

Mesothelioma, a rare and aggressive form of cancer, is primarily attributed to exposure to asbestos, a naturally occurring mineral known for its heat-resistant and insulating properties. Asbestos was once extensively used in various industries, including construction, shipbuilding, and manufacturing. The inhalation or ingestion of microscopic asbestos fibers can lead to their accumulation in the body's mesothelial tissues, triggering cellular changes that may result in the development of mesothelioma. The relationship between asbestos exposure and mesothelioma is well-established, constituting the predominant cause of this challenging disease.

1. Asbestos Exposure:

• Occupational Exposure: Individuals with occupational histories in industries such as construction, insulation, shipbuilding, and asbestos mining face a heightened risk of asbestos exposure. Workers involved in activities that disturb asbestos-containing materials, such as demolition or renovation, are particularly vulnerable.

• Secondary Exposure: While primary exposure occurs in the workplace, secondary exposure can affect individuals who come into contact with asbestos fibers carried on the clothing, skin, or hair of someone directly exposed. This often includes family members of asbestos workers.

2. Other Potential Risk Factors:

• Zeolite Exposure: Some studies suggest a possible association between exposure to zeolites, minerals with chemical similarities to asbestos, and an increased risk of mesothelioma. However, this link is less well-established than the connection with asbestos.

• Radiation Exposure: High-dose radiation therapy, particularly to the chest or abdomen, has been identified as a potential risk factor for mesothelioma. This is more common in individuals who have undergone radiation treatment for other cancers.

• SV40 Virus: Simian Virus 40 (SV40), a virus that contaminated some batches of polio vaccine administered in the late 1950s and early 1960s, has been investigated as a potential cofactor in mesothelioma development. However, the role of SV40 in mesothelioma remains controversial and is not universally accepted.

SYMPTOMS OF MESOTHELIOMA

Recognizing and understanding the symptoms of mesothelioma are crucial for early detection and timely intervention. Here are the common symptoms associated with mesothelioma:

1. Pleural Mesothelioma Symptoms:

• Chest Pain: Persistent and sometimes severe pain in the chest is a common symptom. This can result from the tumor invading the chest wall or affecting the pleura.

• Shortness of Breath: Difficulty breathing and shortness of breath may occur as the tumor grows and puts pressure on the lungs.

• Persistent Cough: A chronic cough that may be accompanied by blood-tinged sputum is a frequent symptom.

• Pleural Effusion: Accumulation of fluid in the pleural cavity can lead to pleural effusion, causing further difficulty breathing.

2. Peritoneal Mesothelioma Symptoms:

• Abdominal Pain: Persistent and often severe pain in the abdominal region is a common symptom.

• Abdominal Swelling: Swelling or a noticeable increase in

abdominal girth may occur due to the accumulation of fluid (ascites).

• Changes in Bowel Habits: Mesothelioma affecting the peritoneum can lead to changes in bowel habits, including constipation or diarrhea.

• Weight Loss: Unexplained and unintentional weight loss is a common symptom of peritoneal mesothelioma.

3. Pericardial Mesothelioma Symptoms:

• Chest Pain: Individuals with pericardial mesothelioma often experience chest pain due to the tumor affecting the pericardium around the heart.

• Irregular Heartbeat: Cardiac symptoms, such as palpitations or uneven heartbeats, may occur.

• Difficulty Breathing: As the tumor affects the pericardium and cardiac function, individuals may experience difficulty breathing.

DIAGNOSIS OF MESOTHELIOMA

Diagnosing mesothelioma is a complex process involving medical history evaluation, imaging studies, and biopsy procedures. Due to the rarity of the disease and the challenges associated with its long latency period, accurate and timely diagnosis is crucial for implementing appropriate treatment strategies. Here are the critical aspects of the diagnostic process for mesothelioma:

1. Medical History and Physical Examination:

• Occupational and Environmental History: A detailed history, including occupational and environmental exposures to asbestos, is critical. Individuals with a history of asbestos exposure, especially in high-risk occupations, are at an increased risk of developing mesothelioma.

• Symptom Assessment: A thorough evaluation of symptoms, such as chest pain, difficulty breathing, abdominal discomfort, or unexplained weight loss, provides valuable insights into potential mesothelioma.

2. Imaging Studies:

• Chest X-ray: Often, during the initial imaging study, a chest X-ray may reveal pleural effusion, thickening of the pleura, or other abnormalities.

• CT Scan (Computed Tomography): CT scans provide

detailed cross-sectional images of the chest or abdomen, helping to identify tumor size, location, and potential spread to nearby structures.

• MRI (Magnetic Resonance Imaging): MRI may be employed for further evaluation, particularly in assessing soft tissue involvement and potential tumor spread.

3. Biopsy Procedures:

• Fine-Needle Aspiration (FNA): A thin needle is used to extract a small tissue sample from the suspicious area. FNA is often employed when the tumor is easily accessible.

• Core Needle Biopsy: This procedure involves a larger needle to obtain a more substantial tissue sample for a more accurate diagnosis.

• Surgical Biopsy: A surgical biopsy may be necessary in cases where FNA or core needle biopsy samples are inconclusive. Depending on the affected area, this can involve video-assisted thoracoscopy (VAT), laparoscopy, or open surgery.

4. Pathological Analysis:

• Histopathology: A microscopic examination of the biopsy tissue is conducted by a pathologist to assess the cellular characteristics, confirming the presence of malignant mesothelioma cells.

• Immunohistochemistry: This technique helps identify specific proteins on the surface of cancer cells, aiding in distinguishing mesothelioma from other cancers.

5. Biomarker Testing:

• Mesothelin Levels: Elevated levels of mesothelin, a protein associated with mesothelioma, may be detected through blood tests. While not definitive for diagnosis, it can support the overall assessment.

6. Staging and Further Evaluation:

• Positron Emission Tomography (PET) Scan: PET scans can help determine the extent of tumor spread and aid in staging.

• Lymph Node Biopsy: To assess whether the cancer has spread to nearby lymph nodes.

STAGES OF MESOTHELIOMA

Mesothelioma staging is a crucial component in determining the extent of the disease and plays a pivotal role in guiding treatment decisions. The staging system helps healthcare professionals assess the spread of the cancer, enabling them to tailor an appropriate and individualized treatment plan. The most commonly used staging system for mesothelioma is the TNM system, which considers the size and extent of the tumor (T), whether the cancer has spread to nearby lymph nodes (N), and if it has metastasized to distant organs (M). Here are the stages of mesothelioma:

Stage I: Localized Disease

• Tumor (T): The cancer is confined to the pleura or peritoneum and may involve one lung or one side of the chest wall (T1).

• Lymph Nodes (N): No lymph node involvement (N0).

• Metastasis (M): No distant metastasis (M0).

• Description: Mesothelioma is localized to the point of origin, making surgical intervention potentially curative at this stage.

Stage II: Advanced Localized Disease

• Tumor (T): The cancer has extended into nearby structures or organs but is still confined to one side of the chest or abdomen (T2).

• Lymph Nodes (N): Limited involvement of nearby lymph nodes (N1).

• Metastasis (M): No distant metastasis (M0).

• Description: The cancer has progressed beyond its original location but remains on one side of the body, allowing for specific treatment options.

Stage III: Regional Spread

• Tumor (T): The cancer has spread further into nearby structures or organs, potentially crossing the midline (T3).

• Lymph Nodes (N): Extensive involvement of nearby lymph nodes (N2).

• Metastasis (M): No distant metastasis (M0).

• Description: Mesothelioma has infiltrated surrounding structures and lymph nodes on the same side of the body, limiting curative treatment options.

Stage IV: Distant Spread

• Tumor (T): The cancer has spread extensively to multiple organs or has invaded distant structures (T4).

• Lymph Nodes (N) may involve remote lymph nodes (N3).

• Metastasis (M): Distant metastasis may be present (M1).

• Description: Mesothelioma has spread widely throughout the body, limiting treatment options to palliative care aimed at managing symptoms and improving quality of life.

TREATMENT OPTIONS

The treatment of mesothelioma often involves a multimodal approach, combining different therapeutic interventions to address the complex nature of the disease. The choice of treatment depends on various factors, including the stage of mesothelioma, the tumor's location, the patient's overall health, and individualized considerations. Here are the standard treatment options for mesothelioma:

1. Surgery:

• Pleurectomy/Decortication (P/D): In this procedure for pleural mesothelioma, the surgeon removes the pleura along with visible tumors but leaves the lung intact. P/D is considered an early-stage disease and aims to reduce symptoms and improve quality of life.

• Extrapleural Pneumonectomy (EPP): This surgical approach involves the removal of the pleura, lung, diaphragm, and sometimes the pericardium. EPP is more extensive and is considered in select cases where cancer has not spread extensively.

• Cytoreductive Surgery with HIPEC: For peritoneal mesothelioma, cytoreductive surgery may be combined with hyperthermic intraperitoneal chemotherapy (HIPEC).

This involves removing visible tumors in the abdomen, followed by heated chemotherapy to kill the remaining cancer cells.

2. Chemotherapy:

• Systemic Chemotherapy: The use of drugs, either orally or intravenously, to kill or slow the growth of cancer cells throughout the body. Common chemotherapy drugs for mesothelioma include pemetrexed and cisplatin.

• Intracavitary Chemotherapy: In some cases, chemotherapy drugs may be administered directly into the chest or abdominal cavity during or after surgery to target residual cancer cells.

3. Radiation Therapy:

• External Beam Radiation: High-dose radiation is directed at the tumor from outside the body. It is often used to shrink tumors, alleviate symptoms, or target residual cancer cells after surgery.

• Intraoperative Radiation Therapy (IORT): Radiation is delivered directly to the tumor site during surgery. This approach allows for precise targeting of cancer cells while sparing surrounding healthy tissues.

4. Immunotherapy:

• Immune Checkpoint Inhibitors: Immunotherapy drugs, such as pembrolizumab and nivolumab, aim to enhance the body's immune response against cancer cells. These drugs target specific proteins that inhibit immune system activity.

• Adoptive Cell Therapy: This emerging approach involves modifying a patient's own immune cells (such as T cells) in a laboratory to enhance their ability to recognize and attack cancer cells before infusing them back into the patient.

5. Targeted Therapy:

• Angiogenesis Inhibitors: These drugs target blood vessel formation, preventing the tumor from receiving nutrients and oxygen. Bevacizumab is an example used in combination with chemotherapy for mesothelioma.

6. Supportive Care:

• Palliative Care: While not a direct treatment for the cancer itself, palliative care focuses on improving the quality of life for individuals with mesothelioma. It addresses symptoms, pain management, and emotional well-being.

CHAPTER TWO

*Importance of Nutrition
in Cancer Treatment*

Nutrition plays a crucial role in the overall well-being and management of cancer, including during treatment. Cancer treatment, whether it involves surgery, chemotherapy, radiation therapy, immunotherapy, or a combination of these, can place significant demands on the body. Proper nutrition is essential to support the body's ability to cope with the physical and metabolic challenges associated with cancer and its treatments. Here is the importance of nutrition in cancer treatment:

1. Maintaining Strength and Energy:

• Cancer treatments can often lead to fatigue and a decline in energy levels. Adequate nutrition provides essential nutrients and calories, helping to sustain energy levels and prevent excessive weight loss.

2. Supporting the Immune System:

• Cancer treatments, particularly chemotherapy, can weaken the immune system. A well-balanced diet with sufficient vitamins, minerals, and antioxidants supports immune function, helping the body better cope with infections and potential complications.

3. Preventing Malnutrition:

• Malnutrition is a common concern during cancer treatment due to factors such as decreased appetite, changes in taste, and treatment-related side effects. Proper nutrition helps prevent malnutrition, which can compromise the body's ability to heal and recover.

4. Managing Treatment Side Effects:

• Nutrition can play a role in managing standard treatment side effects. For example, certain foods may help alleviate nausea, and a well-planned diet can address digestive issues such as constipation or diarrhea.

5. Preserving Lean Body Mass:

• Cancer treatments can lead to muscle wasting and loss of lean body mass. Adequate protein intake is crucial to help maintain muscle mass and promote tissue repair.

6. Enhancing Wound Healing:

• Proper nutrition is essential for wound healing for individuals undergoing surgery as part of their cancer treatment. Nutrients such as protein, vitamins, and minerals play critical roles in the repair and regeneration of tissues.

7. Improving Treatment Tolerance:

• Good nutrition may enhance the tolerability of cancer treatments. Well-nourished individuals may be better equipped to withstand the physical stress of treatments, reducing the risk of treatment delays or interruptions.

8. Addressing Nutrient Deficiencies:

• Cancer patients may experience nutrient deficiencies due to factors such as reduced intake, malabsorption, or increased nutrient needs. Addressing these deficiencies through dietary adjustments or supplements can support overall health.

9. Enhancing Quality of Life:

• Proper nutrition contributes to an improved quality of life during cancer treatment. It can positively impact mood, reduce treatment-related discomfort, and provide a sense of control and well-being.

10. Individualized Nutrition Plans:

• Each person's nutritional needs are unique, and an individualized nutrition plan takes into account factors such as the type of cancer, treatment modalities, overall health, and personal preferences. Working with a registered dietitian can help tailor a plan that meets specific needs.

FOODS TO EAT AS A MESOTHELIOMA PATIENT

A well-balanced and nourishing diet is crucial for individuals with mesothelioma, as it can help support overall health, manage treatment side effects, and enhance the body's ability to cope with the challenges of cancer. While nutritional needs can vary from person to person, here is a guide to foods that may be beneficial for mesothelioma patients:

1. Fruits and Vegetables:

• Rich in vitamins, minerals, and antioxidants, fruits and vegetables support overall health and may help combat inflammation. Choose a variety of colorful options, such as berries, leafy greens, citrus fruits, and cruciferous vegetables.

2. Lean Proteins:

• Protein is essential for preserving muscle mass and promoting tissue repair. Opt for lean protein sources such as poultry, fish, tofu, legumes, and eggs.

3. Whole Grains:

• Whole grains provide a good source of energy and fiber.

Include options like brown rice, quinoa, whole wheat, oats, and whole-grain pasta in your diet.

4. Healthy Fats:

• Incorporate sources of healthy fats, such as avocados, nuts, seeds, and olive oil. These fats provide essential fatty acids and can contribute to a well-rounded diet.

5. Dairy or Dairy Alternatives:

• Dairy products or fortified dairy alternatives are necessary for obtaining calcium and vitamin D, which are essential for bone health. Choose low-fat or non-dairy options if preferred.

6. Hydration:

• Staying well-hydrated is crucial, especially during cancer treatment. Consume plenty of water, herbal teas, and clear broths to prevent dehydration and support overall well-being.

7. Small, Frequent Meals:

• Eating smaller, more frequent meals throughout the day may be easier to manage, especially if treatment side effects such as nausea or changes in appetite are present.

8. High-calorie, Nutrient-Dense Foods:

• Choose calorie-dense foods that pack a nutritional punch, such as nuts, seeds, nut butter, and dried fruits. This can be helpful for maintaining weight and energy levels.

9. Foods to Combat Nausea:

• Ginger, peppermint, and bland foods like crackers or toast may help alleviate nausea. Experiment with smaller, more easily digestible meals and snacks.

10. Individualized Nutrition Plans:

• Work with a registered dietitian or nutritionist to develop a personalized nutrition plan that takes into account your specific needs, preferences, and any treatment-related challenges.

FOODS TO AVOID AS A MESOTHELIOMA PATIENT

For individuals with mesothelioma, paying attention to dietary choices is crucial, especially considering the potential impact of certain foods on treatment side effects and overall well-being. While individual responses to foods can vary, here is a guide to foods that may be advisable to limit or avoid for mesothelioma patients:

1. High-Fat and Fried Foods:

• Foods high in unhealthy fats, such as fried items, processed snacks, and fatty cuts of meat, maybe more complex to digest and can contribute to feelings of discomfort or nausea.

2. Processed and Preservative-Laden Foods:

• Highly processed and preserved foods often contain additives and chemicals that may not be conducive to overall health. Opt for whole, fresh foods whenever possible.

3. Excessive Sugar and Sweets:

• Excessive sugar intake can contribute to inflammation and may impact energy levels. Limit the consumption of sugary snacks, candies, and desserts.

4. Salty Foods:

• High-sodium foods can contribute to fluid retention and may exacerbate issues related to edema or swelling. Be mindful of salt intake and opt for fresh, whole foods over processed items.

5. Caffeine and Stimulants:

• Caffeine and other stimulants can potentially interfere with sleep patterns and exacerbate feelings of anxiety or restlessness. Consider limiting or avoiding caffeinated beverages, especially in the evening.

6. Alcohol:

• Alcohol can have detrimental effects on the liver and may interact with certain medications. It is advisable to limit or abstain from alcohol consumption during cancer treatment.

7. Spicy Foods:

• Spicy foods may contribute to gastrointestinal discomfort, acid reflux, or irritation. If you experience digestive issues, consider limiting the intake of overly spicy foods.

8. Large Meals:

• Eating large meals may contribute to feelings of fullness and discomfort, especially if you are dealing with treatment-related side effects like nausea. Consider smaller, more frequent meals.

9. Dairy Products (if Lactose Intolerant):

• Some individuals may experience lactose intolerance during cancer treatment. If lactose intolerance is an issue, consider lactose-free or dairy alternatives.

10. Gas-Producing Foods:

• Certain foods can contribute to gas and bloating. This may include cruciferous vegetables (broccoli, cauliflower), beans, and carbonated beverages. Experiment with different cooking methods to make these foods more digestible.

11. Individualized Avoidances:

• Pay attention to any specific food aversions or intolerances that may arise during treatment. If certain foods cause discomfort or are unappealing, it's acceptable to avoid them temporarily.

ADDRESSING NUTRITIONAL CHALLENGES DURING TREATMENT

Addressing nutritional challenges is a critical aspect of care for individuals undergoing cancer treatment, including those facing mesothelioma. Nausea and vomiting, loss of appetite, and changes in taste and smell are common issues that can significantly impact a patient's ability to maintain proper nutrition. Effectively managing these challenges requires a personalized and multidisciplinary approach involving healthcare professionals, dietitians, and patients themselves. Here's a guide to addressing nutritional challenges during mesothelioma treatment:

1. Nausea and Vomiting:

• Small, Frequent Meals: Instead of consuming large meals, opt for smaller, more frequent meals to help manage nausea.

• Ginger: Ginger has anti-nausea properties. Consider ginger tea, ginger candies, or ginger-infused foods.

• Avoid Strong Odors: Strong smells can trigger nausea. Opt for bland or cold foods and avoid cooking odorous meals.

• Stay Hydrated: Sip fluids between meals rather than with meals to prevent a feeling of fullness that can worsen nausea.

• Medication: Consult with your healthcare team about anti-nausea medications that may be prescribed to manage symptoms.

2. Loss of Appetite:

• Nutrient-Dense Foods: Choose foods that are nutrient-dense to maximize nutritional intake even with smaller portions.

• High-Calorie Snacks: Incorporate high-calorie snacks such as nuts, seeds, and energy-dense smoothies to boost calorie intake.

• Texture Modifications: Experiment with different textures (soft, crunchy, smooth) to find what is more appealing during periods of reduced appetite.

• Eat Before Treatment: Have a small meal or snack before undergoing treatment to help minimize the impact of treatment-related nausea on appetite.

3. Changes in Taste and Smell:

• Experiment with Flavors: Experiment with different herbs and spices to enhance the flavor of foods without relying heavily on salt.

• Marinades and Sauces: Use flavorful marinades and sauces to make foods more appealing.

• Cold or Room Temperature Foods: Cold or room temperature foods may have milder smells and flavors compared to hot foods.

• Citrus and Tart Flavors: Citrus fruits and tart flavors may be more palatable for individuals experiencing changes in taste.

4. Supplements:

• Nutritional Supplements: In consultation with a healthcare provider or dietitian, consider dietary supplements to ensure adequate intake of essential nutrients.

• Protein Supplements: Protein shakes or supplements may help meet protein requirements during periods of reduced food intake.

5. Hydration:

• Infused Water: Infuse water with fruits or herbs to enhance its flavor, making it more appealing for those with changes in taste.

• Electrolyte-Rich Drinks: Consider electrolyte-rich drinks to stay hydrated, especially if there is a dislike for plain water.

6. Psychosocial Support:

• Emotional Support: Emotional and psychological well-being plays a significant role in appetite and nutritional intake. Seek support from counselors, therapists, or support groups.

• Mealtime Environment: Create a positive and enjoyable mealtime environment, which can contribute to a more pleasant eating experience.

7. Regular Monitoring:

• Regular Assessments: Work closely with a registered

dietitian or nutritionist for routine assessments and adjustments to the nutrition plan based on individual needs and treatment responses.

THE ROLE OF SUPPLEMENTS

Supplements play a role in supporting overall health and well-being, especially for individuals undergoing cancer treatment such as mesothelioma. While obtaining nutrients from a well-balanced diet is essential, certain situations may warrant the use of supplements to address specific needs or deficiencies. Here are the role of supplements, focusing on vitamins and minerals, omega-3 fatty acids, and probiotics:

1. Vitamins and Minerals:

• Importance of Cancer Treatment: Cancer treatments, including surgery, chemotherapy, and radiation therapy, can sometimes lead to nutrient deficiencies. Vitamins and minerals are crucial for various physiological functions, and maintaining adequate levels is vital during the treatment process.

• Common Deficiencies: Common deficiencies during cancer treatment include vitamin D, vitamin B12, iron, and calcium. These deficiencies can affect energy levels, immune function, and bone health.

• Supplementation Considerations: Supplementation is typically recommended based on individual needs and deficiencies. Regular monitoring of blood levels and consultation with healthcare providers or dietitians can guide appropriate supplementation.

2. Omega-3 Fatty Acids:

• Anti-Inflammatory Properties: Omega-3 fatty acids, found in fatty fish (such as salmon and mackerel), flaxseeds, and walnuts, have anti-inflammatory properties. Inflammation is a factor in cancer development and progression, and omega-3s may help mitigate this process.

• Supporting Heart Health: Cancer treatments may impact cardiovascular health, and omega-3 supplementation can contribute to heart health. However, discussing supplementation with healthcare providers is essential, especially if individuals are taking blood-thinning medications.

• Potential Side Effects: High doses of omega-3 supplements may have mild side effects, such as gastrointestinal issues or a fishy aftertaste. Moderation and consultation with healthcare providers are essential.

3. Probiotics:

• Gut Health Support: Probiotics are beneficial bacteria that support gut health. Cancer treatments, particularly antibiotics and specific therapies, can disrupt the balance of gut bacteria. Probiotic supplements or foods like yogurt and fermented products may help restore this balance.

• Immune System Modulation: The gut plays a crucial role in immune system function. Probiotics may help modulate the immune system, potentially supporting overall immune health during cancer treatment.

• Individual Response: Responses to probiotics can vary, and it's essential to introduce them gradually to assess tolerance. It's advisable to consult with healthcare providers before incorporating probiotic supplements, especially for individuals with compromised immune systems.

LIFESTYLE MODIFICATIONS

Lifestyle modifications, including exercise and physical activity, as well as prioritizing sleep and rest, play a vital role in supporting the well-being of individuals undergoing cancer treatment, such as mesothelioma. These modifications can positively impact physical and mental health, enhance treatment outcomes, and contribute to an improved quality of life. Here is a guide to lifestyle modifications during cancer treatment:

A. Exercise and Physical Activity:

1. Benefits during Cancer Treatment:

• Improved Physical Function: Regular exercise can help maintain or improve physical function, including strength, flexibility, and endurance. This is particularly important during and after cancer treatment.

• Enhanced Mental Well-being: Exercise has been shown to reduce anxiety, depression, and fatigue, promoting overall mental well-being.

• Immune System Support: Moderate exercise may help support the immune system, potentially reducing the risk of infections during cancer treatment.

• Management of Treatment Side Effects: Physical activity can help manage common treatment-related side effects, such as fatigue, nausea, and changes in mood.

2. Adaptations based on Individual Capabilities:

• Consultation with Healthcare Team: Before starting or modifying an exercise routine, individuals should consult with their healthcare team to ensure safety, mainly if specific health concerns or treatment-related restrictions exist.

• Tailored Exercise Plans: Work with a certified exercise physiologist or physical therapist to develop a customized exercise plan that takes into account individual capabilities, treatment side effects, and personal preferences.

• Gradual Progression: Start with low-intensity activities and gradually progress based on individual tolerance. This may include activities like walking, gentle stretching, or yoga.

B. Sleep and Rest:

1. Importance of Adequate Sleep:

• Recovery and Healing: Quality sleep is crucial for the body's recovery and healing processes, which are particularly important during cancer treatment.

• Mood Regulation: Adequate sleep supports emotional well-being and helps regulate mood, reducing the impact of stress and anxiety.

• Immune System Function: Sleep plays a vital role in maintaining a healthy immune system, which is essential for individuals undergoing cancer treatment.

• Pain Management: Quality sleep can contribute to better pain management and overall comfort.

2. Strategies for Improving Sleep Quality:

• Establishing a Routine: Create a consistent sleep routine by going to bed and waking up at the same time each day, even on weekends.

• Creating a Restful Environment: Ensure the sleep environment is comfortable, relaxed, and dark. Consider using blackout curtains and minimizing noise disruptions.

• Limiting Stimulants: Avoid stimulants such as caffeine and nicotine close to bedtime, as they can interfere with sleep.

• Mind-Body Techniques: Practice relaxation techniques such as deep breathing, meditation, or gentle yoga to promote relaxation before bedtime.

• Limiting Screen Time: Reduce exposure to screens (phones, computers, TVs) at least an hour before bedtime, as the blue light emitted can disrupt the production of melatonin, a hormone that regulates sleep.

• Consultation with Healthcare Providers: If sleep disturbances persist, discuss them with healthcare providers, who can offer guidance on potential interventions or medications to improve sleep quality.

SAMPLE MEAL PLANS

Below are sample meal plans for seven days, with a focus on providing balanced nutrition and addressing potential challenges associated with cancer treatment:

DAY 1:

Breakfast:

- Scrambled eggs with spinach and tomatoes
- Whole grain toast with avocado
- Fresh fruit (e.g., berries or melon)
- Herbal tea or water

Lunch:

- Grilled chicken or tofu salad with mixed greens, cherry tomatoes, cucumber, and a light vinaigrette dressing
- Quinoa or brown rice on the side
- Greek yogurt with honey

Snack:

- Handful of nuts (e.g., almonds or walnuts)
- Fresh apple slices

Dinner:

- Baked salmon or a plant-based protein option
- Steamed broccoli and carrots
- Sweet potato mash
- Whole grain roll
- Herbal tea or water

DAY 2:

Breakfast:

• Oatmeal with sliced banana, chia seeds, and a drizzle of honey

• Low-fat yogurt

• Green tea or water

Lunch:

• Lentil soup with whole grain crackers

• Mixed green salad with a variety of vegetables

• Fresh fruit (e.g., orange slices)

Snack:

• Hummus with carrot and cucumber sticks

• Whole grain crackers

Dinner:

• Grilled chicken or tempeh with quinoa

• Roasted Brussels sprouts with olive oil and garlic

• Mixed berries for dessert

• Water or herbal tea

DAY 3:

Breakfast:

• Whole grain pancakes with fresh berries and a dollop of Greek yogurt

• Scrambled eggs or tofu scramble

• Herbal tea or water

Lunch:

• Turkey or avocado wrap with whole grain tortilla

• Mixed green salad with a variety of colorful vegetables

• Fresh pineapple chunks

Snack:

• Cottage cheese with sliced peaches

• Handful of almonds

Dinner:

• Stir-fried tofu or shrimp with broccoli, bell peppers, and snap peas

• Brown rice or quinoa

• Baked apples with cinnamon for dessert

• Water or herbal tea

DAY 4:

Breakfast:

• Whole grain toast with peanut butter and banana slices

• Greek yogurt with a sprinkle of granola

• Herbal tea or water

Lunch:

• Quinoa and black bean salad with cherry tomatoes, corn, and avocado

• Grilled chicken or a plant-based protein option

• Fresh strawberries for dessert

Snack:

• Rice cakes with hummus and cherry tomatoes

• Mixed nuts (e.g., pistachios and almonds)

Dinner:

• Baked cod or a vegetarian alternative

• Mashed cauliflower with garlic

• Steamed asparagus

• Sliced mango for a sweet ending

• Water or herbal tea

DAY 5:

Breakfast:

• Smoothie with spinach, banana, berries, Greek yogurt, and a touch of honey

• Whole grain muffin or toast

• Green tea or water

Lunch:

• Whole grain pasta with marinara sauce, grilled vegetables, and lean ground turkey or a plant-based alternative

• Mixed green salad with balsamic vinaigrette

• Sliced kiwi for dessert

Snack:

• Cottage cheese with pineapple chunks

• Whole grain crackers

Dinner:

• Stir-fried tofu or shrimp with snap peas, bell peppers, and brown rice

• Roasted sweet potatoes

• Fresh orange slices

• Water or herbal tea

DAY 6:

Breakfast:

- Scrambled eggs with spinach and feta cheese
- Whole grain English muffin with avocado
- Herbal tea or water

Lunch:

- Chicken or chickpea curry with quinoa
- Steamed broccoli and cauliflower
- Sliced watermelon for dessert

Snack:

- Greek yogurt with honey and a handful of granola
- Mixed berries

Dinner:

- Grilled salmon or a plant-based protein option
- Quinoa salad with cucumber, cherry tomatoes, and mint
- Baked apples with cinnamon for dessert
- Water or herbal tea

DAY 7:

Breakfast:

• Overnight oats are made with rolled oats, chia seeds, and almond milk, topped with sliced strawberries and a drizzle of honey.

• Poached eggs on whole-grain toast

• Herbal tea or water

Lunch:

• Turkey or veggie burger on a whole grain bun with lettuce, tomato, and avocado

• Quinoa salad with mixed vegetables

• Fresh pineapple slices

Snack:

• Smoothie with banana, spinach, almond milk, and a scoop of protein powder

• Handful of mixed nuts

Dinner:

• Baked chicken or tofu with lemon and herbs

• Steamed green beans and carrots

• Brown rice pilaf

• Sliced peaches for dessert

• Water or herbal tea

SAMPLE SHOPPING LIST

A carefully planned list helps ensure that nutritious and easily digestible foods are readily available, making meal preparation more convenient. Here's a comprehensive guide to building a grocery shopping list for individuals navigating mesothelioma treatment:

Proteins:

1. Lean meats (chicken, turkey, fish)

2. Plant-based protein sources (tofu, tempeh, legumes)

3. Eggs

4. Greek yogurt or dairy alternatives

5. Nuts and seeds (almonds, walnuts, chia seeds)

Whole Grains:

1. Quinoa

2. Brown rice

3. Whole grain pasta

4. Oats

5. Whole grain bread or wraps

Fruits:

1. Berries (strawberries, blueberries, raspberries)

2. Citrus fruits (oranges, lemons)

3. Apples

4. Bananas

5. Pineapple or mango

Vegetables:

1. Leafy greens (spinach, kale, lettuce)

2. Cruciferous vegetables (broccoli, cauliflower)

3. Colorful vegetables (bell peppers, tomatoes, carrots)

4. Avocado

5. Sweet potatoes

Dairy or Dairy Alternatives:

1. Low-fat or non-fat milk

2. Greek yogurt or plant-based yogurt

3. Cheese (preferably low-fat options)

Healthy Fats:

1. Olive oil

2. Avocado

3. Nuts and seeds

Frozen Foods:

1. Frozen fruits and vegetables (for convenience)

2. Frozen pre-cooked protein options

Canned or Jarred Items:

1. Canned beans (chickpeas, black beans)

2. Canned tuna or salmon

3. Low-sodium broth or soup

4. Tomato sauce or diced tomatoes (low-sodium)

Grains and Cereals:

1. Whole grain cereal

2. Quinoa or rice cakes

3. Granola

Beverages:

1. Water

2. Herbal teas

3. Freshly squeezed juices (in moderation)

4. Electrolyte-rich drinks (if recommended by healthcare providers)

Snacks:

1. Hummus

2. Whole grain crackers

3. Rice cakes

4. Popcorn (plain, air-popped)

5. Fresh fruit for snacking

Condiments and Seasonings:

1. Herbs and spices

2. Olive oil-based dressings

3. Low-sodium soy sauce or tamari

4. Mustard

5. Honey or maple syrup for natural sweetness

Miscellaneous:

1. Ginger (fresh or ground)

2. Garlic

3. Dark chocolate (for occasional indulgence)

4. Nut butter (peanut butter, almond butter)

Considerations:

• Choose low-sodium or no-added-sugar options when possible.

• Opt for fresh, whole foods over processed items.

• Consider any specific dietary restrictions or preferences.

CHAPTER THREE

Lean Proteins Recipes

Grilled Lemon Rosemary Chicken:

Meal Description: This Grilled Lemon Rosemary Chicken is a light and flavorful dish perfect for a healthy and satisfying meal. The combination of zesty lemon and aromatic rosemary adds a burst of freshness to the tender grilled chicken breast. Serve it alongside your favorite veggies or a crisp salad for a delightful, low-calorie dining experience.

Ingredients:

• Four boneless, skinless chicken breasts

• Two lemons (juiced and zested)

• Two tablespoons fresh rosemary (finely chopped)

• Three tablespoons olive oil

• Salt and pepper to taste

Instructions:

1. Marinate the Chicken:
   a. Combine lemon juice, lemon zest, chopped rosemary, olive oil, salt, and pepper in a bowl.
   b. Place the chicken breasts in a resealable plastic bag or shallow dish.
   c. Pour the marinade over the chicken, ensuring each breast is well-coated.
   d. Seal the bag, cover the dish, and refrigerate for at least 30 minutes to let the flavors infuse.
2. Preheat the Grill:
   e. Preheat your grill to medium-high heat.

3. Grill the Chicken:
   f. Remove the chicken from the marinade, allowing any excess to drip off.
   g. Grill the chicken breasts for approximately 6-8 minutes per side or until they reach an internal temperature of 165°F (74°C) and have a nice char.
4. Rest and Serve:
   h. Allow the grilled chicken to rest for a few minutes before serving to retain its juices.
   i. Serve with additional lemon wedges and a sprinkle of fresh rosemary for garnish.

Nutrition Information (Per Serving):

• Calories: 220

• Protein: 30g

• Carbohydrates: 3g

• Fat: 9g

• Saturated Fat: 1.5g

• Cholesterol: 80mg

• Fiber: 1g

• Sugar: 1g

• Sodium: 350mg

Baked Cod with Garlic and Herbs:

Meal Description: This Baked Cod with Garlic and Herbs is a light and flavorful dish that brings out the natural taste of the cod while infusing it with the richness of garlic and aromatic herbs. The simple preparation makes it an ideal choice for a quick and healthy meal. Pair it with your favorite vegetables or a side of quinoa for a well-balanced dinner.

Ingredients:

- Four cod fillets

- Four cloves garlic (minced)

- Two tablespoons fresh parsley (chopped)

- One tablespoon of fresh dill (chopped)

- Two tablespoons of olive oil

- Salt and pepper to taste

- Lemon wedges for serving

Instructions:

1. Preheat the Oven:
   - Preheat your oven to 375°F (190°C).
2. Prepare the Cod:
   - Pat the cod fillets dry with paper towels.
   - Place the fillets on a lightly greased baking sheet lined with parchment paper.
3. Garlic and Herb Mixture:
   - Combine minced garlic, chopped parsley, chopped dill, olive oil, salt, and pepper in a small bowl. Mix well to create a herb-infused paste.
5. Coat the Cod:
   - Spread the garlic and herb mixture evenly over each cod fillet, ensuring they are well-coated on all sides.
6. Bake the Cod:
   - Bake in the preheated oven for approximately 15-20 minutes or until the cod is opaque and flakes easily with a fork.
7. Broil for Crispiness (Optional):
   - If desired, broil for an additional 2-3 minutes to

achieve a golden brown and slightly crispy top.

8. Serve:

• Remove from the oven and let it rest for a few minutes before serving.

• Garnish with additional fresh herbs and serve with lemon wedges on the side.

Nutrition Information (Per Serving):

• Calories: 180

• Protein: 25g

• Carbohydrates: 2g

• Fat: 8g

• Saturated Fat: 1g

• Cholesterol: 50mg

• Fiber: 0.5g

• Sugar: 0g

• Sodium: 150mg

Turkey and Quinoa Stuffed Bell Peppers:

Meal Description: These Turkey and Quinoa Stuffed Bell Peppers are a nutritious and flavorful option, combining lean ground turkey with quinoa and an assortment of colorful vegetables. Packed with protein and essential nutrients, this dish is satisfying and a well-balanced choice for a wholesome dinner. Serve these stuffed peppers with a side of salad for a complete and healthy meal.

Ingredients:

• Four large bell peppers (any color)

• 1 cup quinoa, cooked according to package instructions

• 1 lb lean ground turkey

- 1 onion, finely chopped

- Two cloves garlic, minced

- One can (14 oz) diced tomatoes, drained

- 1 cup black beans, drained and rinsed

- 1 cup corn kernels (fresh or frozen)

- One teaspoon cumin

- One teaspoon of chili powder

- Salt and pepper to taste

- 1 cup shredded cheese (cheddar or your choice)

- Fresh cilantro for garnish (optional)

Instructions:

1. Preheat the Oven:

- Preheat your oven to 375°F (190°C).

2. Prepare the Bell Peppers:

- Cut the tops off the bell peppers and remove the seeds and membranes. Lightly brush the exterior with olive oil if desired.

3. Cook Quinoa:

- Cook the quinoa according to package instructions and set aside.

4. Cook Turkey and Aromatics:

- In a skillet over medium heat, cook the ground turkey until browned. Add chopped onion and minced garlic, cooking until the onion is softened.

5. Combine Ingredients:

- Combine the cooked turkey mixture in a large bowl with

cooked quinoa, diced tomatoes, black beans, corn, cumin, chili powder, salt, and pepper. Mix well.

6. Stuff the Bell Peppers:

• Stuff each bell pepper with the turkey and quinoa mixture, pressing down gently to pack the filling.

7. Top with Cheese:

• Sprinkle shredded cheese over the top of each stuffed pepper.

8. Bake:

• Place the stuffed peppers in a baking dish and bake for 25-30 minutes or until the peppers are tender.

9. Garnish and Serve:

• Remove from the oven, garnish with fresh cilantro if desired, and serve hot.

Nutrition Information (Per Serving):

• Calories: 350

• Protein: 25g

• Carbohydrates: 35g

• Fat: 12g

• Saturated Fat: 5g

• Cholesterol: 60mg

• Fiber: 6g

• Sugar: 5g

• Sodium: 450mg

Shrimp and Avocado Salad:

Meal Description: This Shrimp and Avocado Salad is a light, refreshing, and protein-packed dish that makes for a perfect lunch or dinner. Succulent shrimp, creamy avocado, and a medley of fresh vegetables come together with a zesty lime dressing, creating a delicious and nutritious salad. Enjoy this vibrant combination of flavors for a satisfying and healthy meal.

Ingredients:

- 1 lb large shrimp, peeled and deveined
- Two avocados, diced
- 1 cup cherry tomatoes, halved
- One cucumber, diced
- 1/4 red onion, thinly sliced
- 1/4 cup fresh cilantro, chopped
- Juice of 2 limes
- Two tablespoons of olive oil
- One teaspoon of honey (optional)
- Salt and pepper to taste
- Mixed salad greens for serving

Instructions:

1. Cook the Shrimp:
   a. In a pot of boiling water, cook the shrimp for 2-3 minutes or until they turn pink and opaque. Drain and set aside to cool.
2. Prepare the Salad Base:
   a. Combine diced avocados, cherry tomatoes, cucumber, red onion, and chopped cilantro in a large bowl.
3. Make the Dressing:
   a. Whisk together lime juice, olive oil, honey

(if using), salt, and pepper in a small bowl to create the dressing.

4. Combine and Toss:
   a. Add the cooled shrimp to the bowl of vegetables.
   b. Drizzle the lime dressing over the shrimp and vegetables.
   c. Gently toss the ingredients until evenly coated with the dressing.

5. Serve:
   a. Arrange a bed of mixed salad greens on serving plates.
   b. Spoon the shrimp and avocado mixture over the greens.

6. Garnish and Enjoy:
   - Garnish with additional cilantro if desired.
   - Serve immediately, and enjoy the vibrant flavors of this delightful shrimp and avocado salad.

Nutrition Information (Per Serving):

- Calories: 300

- Protein: 25g

- Carbohydrates: 14g

- Fat: 18g

- Saturated Fat: 3g

- Cholesterol: 180mg

- Fiber: 7g

- Sugar: 4g

- Sodium: 250mg

Tofu and Vegetable Stir-Fry:

Meal Description: This Tofu and Vegetable Stir-Fry is a delicious and nutritious plant-based dish that showcases the versatility of tofu and the vibrant flavors of assorted vegetables. The quick stir-fry method preserves the freshness and crunchiness of the veggies while allowing the tofu to absorb the savory sauce. Serve over brown rice or noodles for a satisfying and wholesome meal.

Ingredients:

For the Stir-Fry:

• One block (14 oz) of firm tofu, pressed and cubed

• 2 cups broccoli florets

• One red bell pepper, thinly sliced

• One carrot, julienned

• 1 cup snap peas, trimmed

• 1 cup mushrooms, sliced

• Three green onions, sliced

• Two tablespoons of vegetable oil

For the Sauce:

• 1/4 cup soy sauce (low-sodium)

• Two tablespoons of hoisin sauce

• One tablespoon of sesame oil

• One tablespoon of rice vinegar

• One tablespoon of maple syrup or agave nectar

• Two cloves garlic, minced

• One teaspoon of fresh ginger, grated

• One tablespoon cornstarch (optional for thickening)

Instructions:

1. Prepare Tofu:
    i. Press the tofu to remove excess water, then cut it into bite-sized cubes.

2. Make the Sauce:
    i. Whisk together soy sauce, hoisin sauce, sesame oil, rice vinegar, maple syrup, minced garlic, and grated ginger in a bowl. If you prefer a thicker sauce, add cornstarch and whisk until smooth.

3. Stir-Fry Tofu:
    i. Heat vegetable oil in a large skillet or wok over medium-high heat.
    ii. Add tofu cubes and stir-fry until golden brown on all sides. Remove tofu from the pan and set aside.

4. Stir-Fry Vegetables:
    i. In the same pan, add a bit more oil if needed.
    ii. Add broccoli, bell pepper, carrot, snap peas, and mushrooms.
    iii. Stir-fry for 4-5 minutes until vegetables are crisp-tender.

5. Combine Tofu and Vegetables:
    i. Return the tofu to the pan with the stir-fried vegetables.
    ii. Pour the sauce over the tofu and vegetables, tossing everything together until well-coated and heated through.

6. Finish and Serve:

    i. Add sliced green onions and toss for an additional minute.

    ii. Serve the tofu and vegetable stir-fry over brown rice or noodles.

Nutrition Information (Per Serving, excluding rice/noodles):

- Calories: 250

- Protein: 15g

- Carbohydrates: 18g

- Fat: 14g

- Saturated Fat: 2g

- Cholesterol: 0mg

- Fiber: 4g

- Sugar: 7g

- Sodium: 600mg

Greek Yogurt Chicken Wrap:

Meal Description: This Greek Yogurt Chicken Wrap is a flavorful and protein-packed meal that combines tender chicken, crisp vegetables, and a zesty Greek yogurt sauce. Wrapped in a whole-grain tortilla, it's a convenient and delicious option for a satisfying lunch or dinner. The Mediterranean-inspired flavors make this cover both nutritious and refreshing.

Ingredients:

For the Chicken:

- 1 lb boneless, skinless chicken breasts

- 1 tablespoon olive oil

- One teaspoon dried oregano
- One teaspoon of garlic powder
- Salt and pepper to taste
- Juice of 1 lemon

For the Greek Yogurt Sauce:

- 1 cup Greek yogurt
- Two tablespoons fresh dill, chopped
- One tablespoon of lemon juice
- One clove of garlic, minced
- Salt and pepper to taste

For the Wrap:

- Whole-grain tortillas
- One cucumber, thinly sliced
- 1 cup cherry tomatoes, halved
- 1/2 red onion, thinly sliced
- 1 cup mixed salad greens (e.g., spinach, arugula)

Instructions:

1. Prepare the Chicken:
    i. Mix olive oil, dried oregano, garlic powder, salt, pepper, and lemon juice in a bowl.
    ii. Coat chicken breasts with the mixture and let them marinate for at least 15 minutes.
    iii. Grill or pan-cook the chicken until fully cooked, approximately 6-8 minutes per side. Let it rest before

slicing.

2. Make the Greek Yogurt Sauce:

    i. Combine Greek yogurt, chopped dill, lemon juice, minced garlic, salt, and pepper in a small bowl. Mix well to create the sauce.

3. Assemble the Wrap:

    i. Lay out the whole-grain tortillas on a flat surface.

    ii. Spread a generous spoonful of the Greek yogurt sauce on each tortilla.

4. Add the Fillings:

    i. Place sliced grilled chicken in the center of each tortilla.

    ii. Add cucumber slices, cherry tomatoes, red onion, and a handful of mixed salad greens.

5. Wrap it Up:

    i. Fold the sides of the tortilla over the fillings and roll it tightly into a wrap.

6. Serve:

    i. Slice the wraps in half diagonally and serve immediately.

Nutrition Information (Per Serving):

- Calories: 350

- Protein: 30g

- Carbohydrates: 25g

- Fat: 15g

- Saturated Fat: 3g

- Cholesterol: 70mg

- Fiber: 5g

- Sugar: 6g

- Sodium: 450mg

Lentil and Spinach Soup with Lean Turkey:

Meal Description: This Lentil and Spinach Soup with Lean Turkey is a hearty and nutritious option that combines the earthy flavors of lentils, the freshness of spinach, and the lean protein of turkey. Packed with fiber and essential nutrients, this soup is both comforting and wholesome. Enjoy a bowl for a satisfying and nourishing meal.

Ingredients:

For the Soup:

- 1 cup dried green or brown lentils, rinsed

- 1 lb lean ground turkey

- One onion, finely chopped

- Three carrots, peeled and diced

- Three celery stalks, diced

- Four cloves garlic, minced

- One can (14 oz) diced tomatoes, undrained

- 8 cups low-sodium chicken or vegetable broth

- Two teaspoons of ground cumin

- One teaspoon of smoked paprika

- One teaspoon of dried thyme

- Salt and pepper to taste

- 4 cups fresh spinach, chopped

- Juice of 1 lemon

For Garnish (Optional):

- Fresh parsley, chopped

- Grated Parmesan cheese

Instructions:

1. Cook Turkey:
    i. In a large pot, brown the lean ground turkey over medium heat until fully cooked. Drain any excess fat.
2. Sauté Vegetables:
    i. Add chopped onions, carrots, celery, and minced garlic to the pot with the turkey. Sauté until the vegetables are softened.
3. Add Lentils and Spices:
    i. Stir in the rinsed lentils, diced tomatoes (with their juices), cumin, smoked paprika, thyme, salt, and pepper.
4. Pour in Broth:
    i. Pour in the chicken or vegetable broth, and bring the soup to a boil.
5. Simmer:
    i. Reduce the heat to low, cover the pot, and let the soup simmer for 25-30 minutes or until lentils are tender.
6. Add Spinach and Lemon Juice:
    i. Stir in the chopped spinach and lemon juice. Simmer for an additional 5 minutes until the spinach wilts.
7. Adjust Seasoning:

        i. Taste the soup and adjust the seasoning as needed, adding more salt or pepper if desired.

8. Serve:

        i. If desired, ladle the soup into bowls and garnish with fresh parsley or grated Parmesan cheese.

Nutrition Information (Per Serving):

- Calories: 300

- Protein: 25g

- Carbohydrates: 35g

- Fat: 7g

- Saturated Fat: 2g

- Cholesterol: 50mg

- Fiber: 12g

- Sugar: 5g

- Sodium: 600mg

Baked Salmon with Dill and Mustard Glaze:

Meal Description: This Baked Salmon with Dill and Mustard Glaze is a simple yet elegant dish that combines the richness of salmon with the zesty flavors of dill and mustard. The result is a succulent and flavorful main course that's perfect for a healthy and delicious dinner. Serve it with your favorite side dishes for a well-rounded meal.

Ingredients:

For the Salmon:

- Four salmon fillets

- Salt and pepper to taste

- Two tablespoons of olive oil

- One lemon, thinly sliced (for garnish)

For the Dill and Mustard Glaze:

- Two tablespoons of Dijon mustard

- One tablespoon of whole grain mustard

- Two tablespoons fresh dill, chopped

- One tablespoon honey

- One tablespoon of olive oil

- Two cloves garlic, minced

- Zest of 1 lemon

Instructions:

1. Preheat the Oven:
   i. Preheat your oven to 375°F (190°C).
2. Prepare the Salmon:
   i. Pat the salmon fillets dry with paper towels and place them on a baking sheet lined with parchment paper.
3. Season the Salmon:
   i. Season the salmon fillets with salt and pepper to taste.
4. Make the Glaze:
   i. Whisk together Dijon mustard, whole grain mustard, chopped dill, honey, olive oil, minced garlic, and lemon zest in a small bowl.
5. Glaze the Salmon:

      i. Brush the mustard and dill glaze generously over the top of each salmon fillet.

6. Bake:

      i. Bake in the preheated oven for 12-15 minutes or until the salmon is cooked through and flakes easily with a fork.

7. Garnish and Serve:

      i. Garnish the baked salmon with additional fresh dill and lemon slices.

     ii. Serve hot with your favorite side dishes, such as roasted vegetables or quinoa.

Nutrition Information (Per Serving):

- Calories: 300

- Protein: 25g

- Carbohydrates: 5g

- Fat: 18g

- Saturated Fat: 3g

- Cholesterol: 65mg

- Fiber: 1g

- Sugar: 3g

- Sodium: 300mg

CHAPTER FOUR

Fruits and Vegetables recipes

Spinach and Berry Salad with Grilled Turkey:

Meal Description: This Spinach and Berry Salad with Grilled Turkey is a refreshing and nutrient-packed dish that combines the vibrant flavors of fresh berries, crisp spinach, and savory grilled turkey. Topped with a tangy balsamic vinaigrette, this salad is a delightful balance of sweet and savory, making it a perfect choice for a light and satisfying lunch or dinner.

Ingredients:

For the Salad:

- 1 lb turkey breast, thinly sliced and grilled
- 8 cups fresh spinach leaves, washed and dried
- 1 cup strawberries, hulled and sliced
- 1 cup blueberries
- 1/2 cup raspberries
- 1/4 cup sliced almonds, toasted
- 1/4 cup crumbled feta cheese (optional)

For the Balsamic Vinaigrette:

- Three tablespoons balsamic vinegar
- One tablespoon of Dijon mustard
- One clove of garlic, minced
- 1/2 cup extra-virgin olive oil
- Salt and pepper to taste

Instructions:

1. Grill Turkey:

      i. Season the turkey breast with salt and pepper.

      ii. Grill until fully cooked, approximately 6-8 minutes per side. Let it rest before slicing it into thin strips.

2. Prepare the Salad:

      i. Combine fresh spinach leaves, sliced strawberries, blueberries, raspberries, and toasted sliced almonds in a large bowl.

3. Make the Balsamic Vinaigrette:

      i. Whisk together balsamic vinegar, Dijon mustard, minced garlic, salt, and pepper in a small bowl.

      ii. Slowly drizzle in the olive oil while continuing to whisk until the vinaigrette is well combined.

4. Assemble the Salad:

      i. Arrange the grilled turkey strips on top of the salad.

      ii. If using, sprinkle crumbled feta cheese over the salad.

5. Drizzle with Vinaigrette:

      i. Drizzle the balsamic vinaigrette over the salad just before serving.

6. Toss and Serve:

      i. Gently toss the salad to coat the ingredients with the vinaigrette.

      ii. Serve immediately and enjoy the delightful combination of flavors.

Nutrition Information (Per Serving):

- Calories: 400

- Protein: 25g

- Carbohydrates: 20g

- Fat: 25g

- Saturated Fat: 4g

- Cholesterol: 55mg

- Fiber: 8g

- Sugar: 8g

- Sodium: 300mg

Roasted Vegetable Quinoa Bowl:

Meal Description: This Roasted Vegetable Quinoa Bowl is a wholesome and satisfying dish that celebrates the natural flavors of colorful roasted vegetables and nutty quinoa. Packed with nutrients and textures, this bowl is delicious and versatile, allowing you to customize it with your favorite toppings. Enjoy a nourishing and plant-based meal that's easy to prepare.

Ingredients:

For the Roasted Vegetables:

- 2 cups broccoli florets

- One bell pepper, sliced

- One zucchini, sliced

- One carrot, julienned

- One red onion, thinly sliced

- Two tablespoons of olive oil

- One teaspoon of dried thyme

- Salt and pepper to taste

For the Quinoa:

• 1 cup quinoa, rinsed and drained

• 2 cups vegetable broth or water

• Salt to taste

For the Bowl:

• One avocado, sliced

• 1/4 cup hummus

• 1/4 cup crumbled feta cheese (optional)

• Fresh herbs (parsley, cilantro) for garnish

• Lemon wedges for serving

Instructions:

1. Preheat the Oven:
   i. Preheat your oven to 400°F (200°C).
2. Prepare the Roasted Vegetables:
   i. In a large bowl, toss broccoli, bell pepper, zucchini, carrot, and red onion with olive oil, dried thyme, salt, and pepper until evenly coated.
   ii. Spread the vegetables in a single layer on a baking sheet.
   iii. Roast in the preheated oven for 20-25 minutes or until the vegetables are tender and slightly caramelized.
3. Cook the Quinoa:
   i. In a saucepan, combine quinoa and vegetable broth or water.

      ii. Bring to a boil, then reduce heat to low, cover, and simmer for 15-20 minutes or until quinoa is cooked and water is absorbed.

     iii. Fluff with a fork and season with salt.

4. Assemble the Bowl:

      i. Divide the cooked quinoa among serving bowls.

      ii. Top with roasted vegetables, sliced avocado, dollops of hummus, and crumbled feta cheese if using.

5. Garnish and Serve:

      i. Garnish the bowl with fresh herbs and serve with lemon wedges on the side.

Nutrition Information (Per Serving):

- Calories: 400

- Protein: 12g

- Carbohydrates: 50g

- Fat: 18g

- Saturated Fat: 3g

- Cholesterol: 5mg

- Fiber: 10g

- Sugar: 5g

- Sodium: 500mg

Mango, Avocado, and Chicken Lettuce Wraps:

Meal Description: These Mango, Avocado, and Chicken Lettuce Wraps are a delightful combination of sweet, creamy, and savory flavors wrapped in crisp lettuce leaves. With juicy mango, creamy avocado, and seasoned chicken, these wraps make for a refreshing and light meal. Enjoy them as an appetizer or a main course for a burst of tropical goodness.

Ingredients:

For the Chicken:

• 1 lb boneless, skinless chicken breasts

• One tablespoon of olive oil

• One teaspoon of ground cumin

• One teaspoon of smoked paprika

• Salt and pepper to taste

For the Mango Avocado Salsa:

• One ripe mango, diced

• One ripe avocado, diced

• 1/2 red onion, finely chopped

• 1/4 cup fresh cilantro, chopped

• Juice of 2 limes

• Salt and pepper to taste

For the Lettuce Wraps:

• Large lettuce leaves (butter lettuce or iceberg work well)

Instructions:

1. Cook the Chicken:
   i. In a skillet, heat olive oil over medium-high heat.
   ii. Season chicken breasts with ground cumin, smoked paprika,

salt, and pepper.

iii. Cook the chicken until fully cooked, approximately 6-8 minutes per side. Let it rest before slicing it into thin strips.

2. Prepare the Mango Avocado Salsa:

i. Combine diced mango, diced avocado, chopped red onion, chopped cilantro, lime juice, salt, and pepper in a bowl. Mix gently to combine.

3. Assemble the Lettuce Wraps:

i. Place a few slices of the cooked chicken in the center of each lettuce leaf.

ii. Spoon the mango avocado salsa over the chicken.

4. Serve:

i. Arrange the lettuce wraps on a serving platter.

ii. Serve immediately, allowing everyone to assemble their wraps at the table.

5. Optional Additions:

i. Drizzle with a light yogurt or lime crema.

ii. Sprinkle with chopped nuts (e.g., almonds or cashews).

Nutrition Information (Per Serving):

- Calories: 300

- Protein: 25g

- Carbohydrates: 20g

• Fat: 15g

• Saturated Fat: 2g

• Cholesterol: 60mg

• Fiber: 6g

• Sugar: 10g

• Sodium: 400mg

Zucchini Noodles with Tomato and Basil Sauce:

Meal Description: These Zucchini Noodles with Tomato and Basil Sauce are a light and low-carb alternative to traditional pasta, offering a burst of fresh flavors. The zucchini noodles, or "zoodles," are paired with a vibrant tomato and basil sauce, creating a satisfying and nutritious dish. This recipe is perfect for those looking to incorporate more vegetables into their diet without sacrificing taste.

Ingredients:

For the Zucchini Noodles:

• Four medium-sized zucchini, spiralized

• One tablespoon of olive oil

• Salt and pepper to taste

For the Tomato and Basil Sauce:

• Two tablespoons of olive oil

• Three cloves garlic, minced

• One can (28 oz) crushed tomatoes

• One teaspoon dried oregano

• One teaspoon of dried basil

• Salt and pepper to taste

• Red pepper flakes (optional, for heat)

For Garnish:

• Fresh basil leaves, chopped

• Grated Parmesan cheese (optional)

Instructions:

1. Prepare the Zucchini Noodles:
    i. Spiralize the zucchini into noodles using a spiralizer.
    ii. Heat olive oil in a large skillet over medium heat.
    iii. Add the zucchini noodles, season with salt and pepper, and sauté for 3-4 minutes until just tender. Be careful not to overcook, as zucchini noodles can become mushy.
2. Make the Tomato and Basil Sauce:
    i. In a separate saucepan, heat olive oil over medium heat.
    ii. Add minced garlic and sauté until fragrant but not browned.
    iii. Pour in the crushed tomatoes and add dried oregano, dried basil, salt, and pepper.
    iv. Add red pepper flakes to taste if you like a bit of heat.
    v. Simmer the sauce for 15-20 minutes, allowing the flavors to meld.
3. Combine and Serve:
    i. Pour the tomato and basil sauce over the sautéed zucchini noodles.
    ii. Toss gently to coat the noodles in the sauce.

4. Garnish and Enjoy:

    i. Garnish with chopped fresh basil and, if desired, grated Parmesan cheese.

    ii. Serve immediately and enjoy this light and flavorful zucchini noodle dish.

Nutrition Information (Per Serving, without Parmesan):

• Calories: 150

• Protein: 4g

• Carbohydrates: 18g

• Fat: 8g

• Saturated Fat: 1g

• Cholesterol: 0mg

• Fiber: 5g

• Sugar: 10g

• Sodium: 400mg

Citrus Glazed Salmon with Roasted Brussels Sprouts:

Meal Description: This Citrus Glazed Salmon with Roasted Brussels Sprouts is a vibrant and nutritious dish that combines the juiciness of citrus-infused salmon with the earthy flavors of roasted Brussels sprouts. The sweet and tangy citrus glaze adds a delightful twist to the dish, making it a perfect option for a wholesome and flavorful dinner.

Ingredients:

For the Citrus Glazed Salmon:

• Four salmon fillets

- Salt and pepper to taste
- Zest of 1 orange
- Zest of 1 lemon
- 1/4 cup orange juice
- Two tablespoons of lemon juice
- Two tablespoons honey
- Two tablespoons soy sauce (low-sodium)
- Two cloves garlic, minced
- One teaspoon of ginger, grated
- One tablespoon of olive oil

For the Roasted Brussels Sprouts:

- 1 lb Brussels sprouts, trimmed and halved
- Two tablespoons of olive oil
- Salt and pepper to taste
- 1/4 cup grated Parmesan cheese (optional for garnish)

Instructions:

1. Preheat the Oven:
    i. Preheat your oven to 400°F (200°C).
2. Prepare the Citrus Glazed Salmon:
    i. Season the salmon fillets with salt and pepper.
    ii. Whisk together orange zest, lemon zest, orange juice, lemon juice, honey, soy sauce, minced garlic, grated ginger, and olive oil in a bowl.
    iii. Place the salmon fillets in a

shallow dish and pour half of the citrus glaze over them. Let them marinate for at least 15 minutes.

3. Roast the Brussels Sprouts:

    i. Toss Brussels sprouts with olive oil, salt, and pepper on a baking sheet.

    ii. Roast in the preheated oven for 20-25 minutes or until the Brussels sprouts are golden brown and crispy on the edges.

4. Bake the Salmon:

    i. Place the marinated salmon fillets on a separate baking sheet.

    ii. Bake in the preheated oven for 12-15 minutes or until the salmon is cooked through and flakes easily.

5. Glaze the Salmon:

    i. During the last few minutes of baking, brush the remaining citrus glaze over the salmon fillets.

6. Serve:

    i. Arrange the roasted Brussels sprouts on a serving platter.

    ii. Place the citrus-glazed salmon on top.

    iii. Optional: Garnish with grated Parmesan cheese.

Nutrition Information (Per Serving):

- Calories: 400

- Protein: 30g

- Carbohydrates: 25g

- Fat: 20g

- Saturated Fat: 4g

- Cholesterol: 80mg

- Fiber: 6g

- Sugar: 15g

- Sodium: 600mg

Watermelon and Feta Salad with Mint:

Meal Description: This Watermelon and Feta Salad with Mint is a refreshing and vibrant dish that combines the sweetness of watermelon with the savory notes of feta cheese, all brought together by the aromatic freshness of mint. This salad perfectly balances flavors, making it an ideal side dish for summer gatherings or a light and hydrating snack.

Ingredients:

For the Salad:

- 4 cups cubed watermelon, seedless

- 1 cup crumbled feta cheese

- 1/2 red onion, thinly sliced

- 1/2 cup fresh mint leaves, torn or chopped

For the Dressing:

- Two tablespoons extra-virgin olive oil

- One tablespoon of balsamic vinegar

- One teaspoon honey

- Salt and pepper to taste

Instructions:

    1. Prepare the Salad:

      i. Combine cubed watermelon, crumbled feta cheese, thinly sliced red onion, and fresh mint leaves in a large bowl.

2. Make the Dressing:

      i. Whisk together extra-virgin olive oil, balsamic vinegar, honey, salt, and pepper in a small bowl.

3. Drizzle and Toss:

      i. Drizzle the dressing over the watermelon and feta mixture.

      ii. Gently toss the ingredients to coat evenly with the dressing.

4. Chill (Optional):

      i. For enhanced flavor, you can refrigerate the salad for 15-30 minutes before serving.

5. Serve:

      i. Transfer the salad to a serving dish or individual plates.

      ii. Garnish with additional mint leaves if desired.

6. Optional Additions:

      i. Add a handful of arugula or baby spinach for a peppery or leafy element.

      ii. Sprinkle with a handful of toasted pine nuts or chopped pistachios for added crunch.

Nutrition Information (Per Serving):

• Calories: 200

• Protein: 8g

- Carbohydrates: 20g

- Fat: 12g

- Saturated Fat: 6g

- Cholesterol: 30mg

- Fiber: 2g

- Sugar: 15g

- Sodium: 300mg

Broccoli and Cauliflower Casserole with Cheese:

Meal Description: This Broccoli and Cauliflower Casserole with Cheese is a comforting and flavorful dish that combines two cruciferous vegetables with a rich and creamy cheese sauce. Baked to golden perfection, this casserole is a satisfying side dish or a vegetarian main course that's perfect for gatherings or family dinners.

Ingredients:

For the Casserole:

- 4 cups broccoli florets

- 4 cups cauliflower florets

- Two tablespoons of olive oil

- Salt and pepper to taste

For the Cheese Sauce:

- Three tablespoons unsalted butter

- Three tablespoons of all-purpose flour

- 2 cups milk

- 2 cups shredded sharp cheddar cheese

- 1/2 teaspoon garlic powder

- 1/2 teaspoon onion powder

• Salt and pepper to taste

For the Topping:

• 1 cup breadcrumbs

• Two tablespoons melted butter

• 1/4 cup grated Parmesan cheese

Instructions:

1. Preheat the Oven:
    i. Preheat your oven to 375°F (190°C).
2. Prepare the Vegetables:
    i. Toss broccoli and cauliflower florets in a large bowl with olive oil, salt, and pepper until evenly coated.
    ii. Spread the vegetables in a single layer in a baking dish.
3. Roast the Vegetables:
    i. Roast in the preheated oven for 20-25 minutes or until the vegetables are slightly tender and have some caramelized edges.
4. Make the Cheese Sauce:
    i. In a saucepan, melt butter over medium heat.
    ii. Stir in flour to create a roux and cook for 1-2 minutes until lightly golden.
    iii. Gradually whisk in milk to avoid lumps.
    iv. Continue to whisk until the sauce thickens.

     v. Reduce heat to low and add shredded cheddar cheese, garlic powder, onion powder, salt, and pepper. Stir until the cheese is melted and the sauce is smooth.

5. Combine Vegetables and Cheese Sauce:
    i. Pour the cheese sauce over the roasted broccoli and cauliflower, ensuring even coverage.

6. Make the Topping:
    i. Combine breadcrumbs, melted butter, and grated Parmesan cheese in a small bowl.

7. Top and Bake:
    i. Sprinkle the breadcrumb mixture evenly over the cheese-covered vegetables.
    ii. Bake in the preheated oven for an additional 15-20 minutes or until the casserole is bubbly and the topping is golden brown.

8. Serve:
    i. Allow the casserole to cool for a few minutes before serving.

Nutrition Information (Per Serving):

• Calories: 300

• Protein: 12g

• Carbohydrates: 20g

• Fat: 20g

• Saturated Fat: 10g

• Cholesterol: 45mg

- Fiber: 5g

- Sugar: 5g

- Sodium: 400mg

Greek Salad with Shrimp:

Meal Description: This Greek Salad with Shrimp is a light and flavorful dish that combines the vibrant colors and tastes of a classic Greek salad with the addition of succulent grilled shrimp. Packed with fresh vegetables, feta cheese, olives, and a zesty vinaigrette, this salad offers a delightful and satisfying meal that's perfect for a healthy lunch or dinner.

Ingredients:

For the Shrimp:

- 1 lb large shrimp, peeled and deveined

- Two tablespoons olive oil

- Two cloves garlic, minced

- One teaspoon dried oregano

- Salt and pepper to taste

- Juice of 1 lemon

For the Salad:

- 4 cups mixed salad greens (lettuce, spinach, arugula)

- One cucumber, sliced

- 1 cup cherry tomatoes, halved

- 1/2 red onion, thinly sliced

- 1/2 cup Kalamata olives, pitted

- 1/2 cup crumbled feta cheese

- 1/4 cup fresh mint leaves, chopped

For the Vinaigrette:

• 1/4 cup extra-virgin olive oil

• Two tablespoons red wine vinegar

• One teaspoon Dijon mustard

• 1 teaspoon honey

• Salt and pepper to taste

Instructions:

1. Marinate and Grill the Shrimp:
    i. Combine shrimp with olive oil, minced garlic, dried oregano, salt, pepper, and lemon juice in a bowl.
    ii. Let the shrimp marinate for at least 15 minutes.
    iii. Grill the shrimp over medium-high heat for 2-3 minutes per side or until opaque and cooked through.
2. Prepare the Salad:
    i. Combine mixed greens, sliced cucumber, cherry tomatoes, thinly sliced red onion, Kalamata olives, crumbled feta cheese, and chopped mint leaves in a large salad bowl.
3. Make the Vinaigrette:
    i. Whisk together extra-virgin olive oil, red wine vinegar, Dijon mustard, honey, salt, and pepper in a small bowl.
4. Assemble the Salad:
    i. Drizzle the vinaigrette over the salad ingredients.
    ii. Toss the salad gently to coat

everything with the dressing.

5. Top with Grilled Shrimp:

i. Arrange the grilled shrimp on top of the salad.

6. Serve:

i. Serve immediately, and enjoy this Mediterranean-inspired salad with a perfect balance of flavors.

Nutrition Information (Per Serving):

• Calories: 350

• Protein: 25g

• Carbohydrates: 15g

• Fat: 20g

• Saturated Fat: 6g

• Cholesterol: 150mg

• Fiber: 4g

• Sugar: 7g

• Sodium: 600mg

CHAPTER FIVE

Healthy Fats recipes

Avocado and Chickpea Salad:

Meal Description: This Avocado and Chickpea Salad is a light and nutritious dish that combines the creamy texture of ripe avocados with the protein-packed goodness of chickpeas. Tossed with fresh vegetables and a zesty dressing, this salad is delicious and a quick and satisfying option for a healthy lunch or side dish.

Ingredients:

For the Salad:

• Two ripe avocados, diced

• One can (15 oz) chickpeas, drained and rinsed

• 1 cup cherry tomatoes, halved

• One cucumber, diced

• 1/4 cup red onion, finely chopped

• 1/4 cup fresh cilantro or parsley, chopped

For the Dressing:

• Two tablespoons extra-virgin olive oil

• One tablespoon of red wine vinegar

• One clove of garlic, minced

• One teaspoon of Dijon mustard

• Salt and pepper to taste

• Optional: Lemon juice for added freshness

Instructions:

    1. Prepare the Salad Ingredients:

        i. Combine diced avocados,

chickpeas, cherry tomatoes, diced cucumber, chopped red onion, and fresh cilantro or parsley in a large salad bowl.

2. Make the Dressing:
    i. Whisk together extra-virgin olive oil, red wine vinegar, minced garlic, Dijon mustard, salt, and pepper in a small bowl.
    ii. Optionally, add a squeeze of lemon juice for an extra citrusy kick.

3. Assemble the Salad:
    i. Drizzle the dressing over the salad ingredients.
    ii. Gently toss the salad to ensure it is even coated with the dressing.

4. Serve:
    i. Serve the Avocado and Chickpea Salad immediately as a refreshing and satisfying meal or side dish.

5. Optional Additions:
    i. Add crumbled feta cheese for a creamy and tangy element.
    ii. Toss in some olives for a salty flavor.
    iii. Include diced bell peppers or radishes for extra crunch.

Nutrition Information (Per Serving):

• Calories: 300

• Protein: 8g

• Carbohydrates: 25g

- Fat: 20g

- Saturated Fat: 3g

- Cholesterol: 0mg

- Fiber: 10g

- Sugar: 5g

- Sodium: 400mg

Salmon and Avocado Sushi Bowl:

Meal Description: This Salmon and Avocado Sushi Bowl brings the flavors of sushi to a convenient and deconstructed form. Packed with fresh salmon, creamy avocado, and a medley of vegetables, this bowl offers the delicious taste of sushi without the need for rolling. Drizzled with a savory soy-based dressing, it's a satisfying and healthy meal option.

Ingredients:

For the Sushi Bowl:

- 2 cups sushi rice, cooked and seasoned with rice vinegar

- 1 lb fresh salmon, sushi-grade, thinly sliced

- Two ripe avocados, sliced

- One cucumber, julienned

- One carrot, julienned

- 1/4 cup pickled ginger

- 1/4 cup edamame beans, steamed

- Sesame seeds for garnish

- Nori (seaweed) strips, shredded for topping

For the Dressing:

- Three tablespoons soy sauce

• One tablespoon of sesame oil

• One tablespoon of rice vinegar

• One teaspoon honey

• One teaspoon of grated ginger

• One clove of garlic, minced

Instructions:

1. Prepare the Sushi Bowl Ingredients:
    i. Cook sushi rice according to package instructions and season with rice vinegar.
    ii. Arrange the cooked rice in serving bowls.
2. Slice and Arrange the Salmon:
    i. Thinly slice the sushi-grade salmon.
    ii. Arrange the sliced salmon on top of the sushi rice.
3. Add Vegetables:
    i. Place sliced avocados, julienned cucumber, and julienned carrot around the salmon.
4. Top with Garnishes:
    i. Sprinkle sesame seeds over the bowl.
    ii. Add shredded nori strips for a hint of seaweed flavor.
    iii. Arrange pickled ginger and steamed edamame beans.
5. Make the Dressing:
    i. Whisk together soy sauce, sesame oil, rice vinegar, honey, grated

ginger, and minced garlic in a small bowl.

6. Drizzle with Dressing:
    i. Drizzle the dressing over the sushi bowl, ensuring it coats the ingredients evenly.

7. Serve:
    i. Serve the Salmon and Avocado Sushi Bowl immediately, mixing the ingredients together before enjoying.

8. Optional Additions:
    i. Include radish slices or watermelon radishes for extra crunch.
    ii. Add a sprinkle of furikake (Japanese seasoning) for additional flavor.
    iii. Top with a dollop of wasabi or a drizzle of spicy mayo for heat.

Nutrition Information (Per Serving):

• Calories: 400

• Protein: 25g

• Carbohydrates: 50g

• Fat: 15g

• Saturated Fat: 2g

• Cholesterol: 40mg

• Fiber: 6g

• Sugar: 4g

• Sodium: 800mg

Walnut and Pomegranate Quinoa Salad:

Meal Description: This Walnut and Pomegranate Quinoa Salad is a vibrant and nutritious dish that combines the earthy flavor of quinoa with the crunch of walnuts and the sweet burst of pomegranate seeds. Tossed with a lemony vinaigrette, this salad is visually appealing and a delicious and wholesome option for a light lunch or a flavorful side dish.

Ingredients:

For the Salad:

• 1 cup quinoa, rinsed and cooked according to package instructions

• 1 cup pomegranate seeds

• 1/2 cup chopped walnuts, toasted

• One cucumber, diced

• 1/4 cup red onion, finely chopped

• 1/4 cup fresh parsley, chopped

• Feta cheese, crumbled (optional)

For the Lemon Vinaigrette:

• Three tablespoons extra-virgin olive oil

• Juice of 1 lemon

• One teaspoon of Dijon mustard

• One teaspoon honey

• Salt and pepper to taste

Instructions:

    1. Prepare the Quinoa:

        i. Cook quinoa according to package

instructions. Once cooked, fluff it with a fork and let it cool to room temperature.

2. Toast the Walnuts:

    i. In a dry skillet over medium heat, toast the chopped walnuts for 3-5 minutes or until fragrant. Be careful not to burn them.

3. Assemble the Salad:

    i. Combine cooked quinoa, pomegranate seeds, toasted walnuts, diced cucumber, chopped red onion, and fresh parsley in a large bowl.

    ii. If using, sprinkle crumbled feta cheese over the salad.

4. Make the Lemon Vinaigrette:

    i. Whisk together extra-virgin olive oil, lemon juice, Dijon mustard, honey, salt, and pepper in a small bowl.

5. Drizzle and Toss:

    i. Drizzle the lemon vinaigrette over the salad.

    ii. Gently toss the ingredients to ensure an even coating with the dressing.

6. Chill (Optional):

    i. For enhanced flavors, refrigerate the salad for at least 30 minutes before serving.

7. Serve:

    i. Serve the Walnut and Pomegranate

Quinoa Salad chilled or at room temperature.

8. Optional Additions:
    i. Add arugula or spinach leaves for an extra leafy element.
    ii. Include diced apple or pear for a touch of sweetness and crunch.
    iii. Garnish with additional fresh herbs like mint or basil.

Nutrition Information (Per Serving):

• Calories: 350

• Protein: 10g

• Carbohydrates: 40g

• Fat: 18g

• Saturated Fat: 2g

• Cholesterol: 0mg

• Fiber: 6g

• Sugar: 8g

• Sodium: 150mg

Olive Oil and Herb Marinated Grilled Chicken:

Meal Description: This Olive Oil and Herb Marinated Grilled Chicken is a flavorful and juicy dish that highlights the natural taste of the chicken with a blend of herbs and the richness of olive oil. The marinade infuses the chicken with savory and aromatic flavors, and grilling adds a delicious smokiness. Serve this grilled chicken as a main course alongside your favorite sides for a delightful meal.

Ingredients:

For the Marinade:

- Four boneless, skinless chicken breasts
- 1/4 cup extra-virgin olive oil
- Two tablespoons of fresh lemon juice
- Two cloves garlic, minced
- One teaspoon dried oregano
- One teaspoon of dried thyme
- One teaspoon of dried rosemary
- One teaspoon paprika
- Salt and black pepper to taste

For Garnish (Optional):

- Fresh parsley, chopped
- Lemon wedges

Instructions:

1. Prepare the Marinade:
    i. Whisk together extra-virgin olive oil, fresh lemon juice, minced garlic, dried oregano, dried thyme, rosemary, paprika, salt, and black pepper in a bowl.
2. Marinate the Chicken:
    i. Place the chicken breasts in a zip-top bag or shallow dish.
    ii. Pour the marinade over the chicken, ensuring all pieces are well coated.
    iii. Seal the bag or cover the dish and refrigerate for at least 30 minutes, or preferably, marinate for 4-6 hours or overnight for maximum

flavor.

3. Preheat the Grill:
     i. Preheat your grill to medium-high heat.

4. Grill the Chicken:
     i. Remove the chicken from the marinade and let any excess drip off.
     ii. Grill the chicken breasts for 6-8 minutes per side or until the internal temperature reaches 165°F (74°C) and the chicken is no longer pink in the center.

5. Rest and Garnish:
     i. Let the grilled chicken rest for a few minutes before slicing.
     ii. Garnish with fresh chopped parsley and serve with lemon wedges on the side.

6. Serve:
     i. Serve the Olive Oil and Herb Marinated Grilled Chicken as a main course with your favorite sides, such as roasted vegetables, quinoa, or a green salad.

7. Optional Serving Suggestions:
     i. Pair with a side of tzatziki sauce for a Mediterranean twist.
     ii. Serve over a bed of couscous or orzo for a complete meal.

Nutrition Information (Per Serving):

• Calories: 250

• Protein: 30g

• Carbohydrates: 2g

• Fat: 14g

• Saturated Fat: 2g

• Cholesterol: 80mg

• Fiber: 1g

• Sugar: 0g

• Sodium: 350mg

Almond-Crusted Baked Tilapia:

Meal Description: This Almond-Crusted Baked Tilapia is a light and flavorful dish that combines the mild taste of tilapia with a crunchy almond crust. Baking the tilapia ensures a healthy and easy preparation while preserving the fish's natural flavors. Serve this dish with a side of fresh vegetables or a light salad for a delicious and nutritious meal.

Ingredients:

For the Almond Crust:

• Four tilapia fillets

• 1 cup almonds, finely chopped or ground

• 1/4 cup breadcrumbs (optional for added texture)

• Two tablespoons fresh parsley, chopped

• One teaspoon of lemon zest

• 1/2 teaspoon garlic powder

• Salt and pepper to taste

• Two tablespoons olive oil

For Garnish (Optional):

- Lemon wedges

- Fresh parsley, chopped

Instructions:

1. Preheat the Oven:
    i. Preheat your oven to 400°F (200°C).

2. Prepare the Almond Crust:
    i. In a shallow dish, combine finely chopped or ground almonds, breadcrumbs (if using), chopped fresh parsley, lemon zest, garlic powder, salt, and pepper.

3. Coat the Tilapia:
    i. Brush each tilapia fillet with olive oil, ensuring both sides are coated.

4. Coat with Almond Mixture:
    i. Press each tilapia fillet into the almond mixture, coating both sides evenly. Press the almonds onto the fish to ensure they adhere.

5. Arrange on Baking Sheet:
    i. Place the almond-crusted tilapia fillets on a baking sheet lined with parchment paper or lightly greased.

6. Bake:
    i. Bake in the preheated oven for 12-15 minutes or until the tilapia is cooked through and the almond crust is golden brown and crispy.

7. Garnish and Serve:
    i. Garnish with fresh chopped

parsley and lemon wedges if desired.

ii. Serve the Almond-Crusted Baked Tilapia hot with your favorite sides.

8. Optional Serving Suggestions:

i. Serve over a bed of quinoa or brown rice.

ii. Pair with a side of steamed asparagus or roasted vegetables.

Nutrition Information (Per Serving):

• Calories: 300

• Protein: 30g

• Carbohydrates: 8g

• Fat: 18g

• Saturated Fat: 2g

• Cholesterol: 60mg

• Fiber: 4g

• Sugar: 1g

• Sodium: 100mg

Avocado and Shrimp Lettuce Wraps:

Meal Description: These Avocado and Shrimp Lettuce Wraps are a light and refreshing option that combines succulent shrimp with creamy avocado, crisp vegetables, and a zesty dressing. Wrapped in fresh lettuce leaves, these wraps make a healthy and satisfying meal perfect for a quick lunch or a delightful appetizer.

Ingredients:

For the Shrimp:

- 1 lb large shrimp, peeled and deveined
- One tablespoon of olive oil
- One teaspoon of smoked paprika
- 1/2 teaspoon cumin
- Salt and pepper to taste
- Juice of 1 lime

For the Lettuce Wraps:

- One head of iceberg or butter lettuce, leaves separated

For the Filling:

- Two ripe avocados, diced
- 1 cup cherry tomatoes, halved
- 1/2 red onion, finely chopped
- 1/4 cup fresh cilantro, chopped
- One jalapeño, finely chopped (optional for heat)

For the Dressing:

- Three tablespoons olive oil
- Two tablespoons of fresh lime juice
- One teaspoon honey
- Salt and pepper to taste

Instructions:

1. Prepare the Shrimp:
   i. Toss the shrimp with olive oil, smoked paprika, cumin, salt, pepper, and lime juice in a bowl.
   ii. Let the shrimp marinate for 10-15 minutes.

2. Cook the Shrimp:
   i. Heat a skillet over medium-high heat.
   ii. Cook the shrimp for 2-3 minutes per side or until they are opaque and cooked through.
3. Prepare the Lettuce Wraps:
   i. Wash and separate the leaves of iceberg or butter lettuce.
4. Assemble the Filling:
   i. Combine diced avocados, halved cherry tomatoes, finely chopped red onion, chopped cilantro, and, if desired, finely chopped jalapeño.
5. Make the Dressing:
   i. Whisk together olive oil, fresh lime juice, honey, salt, and pepper in a small bowl.
6. Assemble the Wraps:
   i. Place a spoonful of the avocado and shrimp filling onto each lettuce leaf.
   ii. Drizzle the dressing over the filling.
7. Serve:
   i. Serve the Avocado and Shrimp Lettuce Wraps immediately, and enjoy this light and flavorful dish.
8. Optional Additions:
   i. Top with crumbled feta or queso fresco for a tangy twist.
   ii. Sprinkle with chopped green onions for extra freshness.

iii. Add a dash of hot sauce for a spicy kick.

Nutrition Information (Per Serving):

• Calories: 300

• Protein: 20g

• Carbohydrates: 15g

• Fat: 18g

• Saturated Fat: 3g

• Cholesterol: 150mg

• Fiber: 6g

• Sugar: 5g

• Sodium: 200mg

Chia Seed Pudding with Berries:

Meal Description: This Chia Seed Pudding with Berries is a wholesome and nutritious dessert or breakfast option. Chia seeds absorb liquid to create a pudding-like consistency. When combined with creamy coconut milk and topped with fresh berries, it becomes a delicious and satisfying treat that's rich in fiber and omega-3 fatty acids.

Ingredients:

For the Chia Seed Pudding:

• 1/4 cup chia seeds

• 1 cup coconut milk (or any milk of your choice)

• One tablespoon of maple syrup or honey

• 1/2 teaspoon vanilla extract

For Topping:

• Mixed berries (strawberries, blueberries, raspberries)

• Sliced almonds or shredded coconut (optional)

Instructions:

1. Prepare the Chia Seed Pudding:
    i. Combine chia seeds, coconut milk, maple syrup or honey, and vanilla extract in a bowl.
    ii. Whisk the mixture thoroughly to ensure the chia seeds are well distributed.
2. Chill:
    i. Cover the bowl and refrigerate the chia seed mixture for at least 4 hours or overnight. This allows the chia seeds to absorb the liquid and create a pudding-like consistency.
3. Stir Before Serving:
    i. Before serving, stir the chia seed pudding well to break up any clumps and achieve a smooth texture.
4. Assemble:
    i. Divide the chia seed pudding into serving bowls or glasses.
5. Top with Berries:
    i. Arrange a generous amount of mixed berries on top of each serving.
6. Optional Garnish:
    i. Sprinkle sliced almonds or shredded coconut on top for added texture and flavor.
7. Serve:

i. Serve the Chia Seed Pudding with Berries immediately and enjoy a delightful and nutritious treat.

8. Optional Variations:

i. Add a dollop of Greek yogurt for a creamier texture.

ii. Drizzle with a bit more maple syrup or honey for extra sweetness.

iii. Include a cinnamon pinch or a citrus juice splash for flavor variation.

Nutrition Information (Per Serving):

• Calories: 250

• Protein: 5g

• Carbohydrates: 20g

• Fat: 16g

• Saturated Fat: 12g

• Cholesterol: 0mg

• Fiber: 10g

• Sugar: 8g

• Sodium: 20mg

Pesto Zucchini Noodles with Pine Nuts:

Meal Description: These Pesto Zucchini Noodles with Pine Nuts are a light and vibrant alternative to traditional pasta, offering a burst of fresh flavors. Spiralized zucchini noodles are tossed in a basil pesto sauce and topped with toasted pine nuts for a quick, healthy, and delicious meal.

Ingredients:

For the Pesto:

- 2 cups fresh basil leaves, packed
- 1/2 cup grated Parmesan cheese
- 1/3 cup pine nuts, toasted
- Two cloves garlic peeled
- 1/2 cup extra-virgin olive oil
- Salt and pepper to taste
- Juice of 1 lemon (optional)

For the Zucchini Noodles:

- Four medium zucchini, spiralized
- One tablespoon olive oil
- Salt and pepper to taste

For Topping:

- 1/4 cup pine nuts, toasted
- Grated Parmesan cheese
- Fresh basil leaves for garnish

Instructions:

1. Prepare the Pesto:
    i. Combine fresh basil, grated Parmesan cheese, toasted pine nuts, and peeled garlic in a food processor.
    ii. Pulse until ingredients are finely chopped.
    iii. With the food processor running, slowly drizzle in the olive oil until the pesto reaches a smooth

consistency.

    iv. Season with salt and pepper to taste. Add lemon juice if desired for brightness.

2. Toast Pine Nuts:

    i. In a dry skillet over medium heat, toast pine nuts until golden brown. Be careful not to burn them. Set aside for topping.

3. Spiralize Zucchini:

    i. Use a spiralizer to turn the zucchini into noodles. If you don't have a spiralizer, you can use a vegetable peeler to create thin ribbons.

4. Cook Zucchini Noodles:

    i. In a large skillet, heat olive oil over medium heat.

    ii. Add the zucchini noodles and sauté for 2-3 minutes or until they are heated. Be cautious not to overcook, as zucchini noodles can become watery.

5. Toss with Pesto:

    i. Add the prepared pesto to the zucchini noodles and toss until evenly coated.

6. Serve:

    i. Divide the Pesto Zucchini Noodles among serving plates.

    ii. Top with toasted pine nuts, grated Parmesan cheese, and fresh basil leaves for garnish.

7. Enjoy:

      i. Serve immediately and enjoy this light and flavorful dish.

8. Optional Additions:

      i. Toss in cherry tomatoes or sun-dried tomatoes for a burst of sweetness.

      ii. Include grilled chicken or shrimp for added protein.

      iii. Mix in baby spinach or arugula for extra greens.

Nutrition Information (Per Serving):

- Calories: 300

- Protein: 8g

- Carbohydrates: 10g

- Fat: 25g

- Saturated Fat: 4g

- Cholesterol: 5mg

- Fiber: 5g

- Sugar: 4g

- Sodium: 150mg

CHAPTER SIX

Whole Grains recipes

Quinoa and Vegetable Stir-Fry with Tofu:

Meal Description: This Quinoa and Vegetable Stir-Fry with Tofu is a wholesome and flavorful dish that combines protein-packed tofu with a variety of colorful vegetables and nutty quinoa. Tossed in a savory stir-fry sauce, this meal offers a perfect balance of textures and tastes, making it a satisfying and nutritious option for lunch or dinner.

Ingredients:

For the Stir-Fry:

• 1 cup quinoa, rinsed

• 2 cups water or vegetable broth

• One block of firm tofu pressed and cubed

• Two tablespoons soy sauce or tamari

• One tablespoon of sesame oil

• One tablespoon of vegetable oil

• 3 cups mixed vegetables (broccoli, bell peppers, snap peas, carrots), chopped

• Three green onions, sliced

• Two cloves garlic, minced

• One tablespoon of fresh ginger, grated

• Sesame seeds for garnish (optional)

For the Stir-Fry Sauce:

• Three tablespoons soy sauce or tamari

• Two tablespoons of hoisin sauce

• One tablespoon of rice vinegar

• One tablespoon of maple syrup or honey

• One teaspoon of cornstarch mixed with two tablespoons water (cornstarch slurry)

Instructions:

1. Cook Quinoa:
    i.   In a saucepan, combine quinoa and water or vegetable broth.
    ii. Bring to a boil, then reduce heat, cover, and simmer for 15-20 minutes or until quinoa is cooked and liquid is absorbed.

2. Press and Marinate Tofu:
    i.   Press the tofu to remove excess water, then cut it into cubes.
    ii. Marinate the tofu cubes in soy sauce and sesame oil in a bowl. Let it marinate for at least 15 minutes.

3. Prepare Stir-Fry Sauce:
    i.   Whisk together soy sauce, hoisin sauce, rice vinegar, maple syrup or honey, and the cornstarch slurry in a small bowl. Set aside.

4. Sauté Tofu:
    i.   Heat vegetable oil in a large skillet or wok over medium-high heat.
    ii. Add the marinated tofu cubes and cook until golden brown on all sides. Remove tofu from the pan and set aside.

5. Stir-Fry Vegetables:
    i.   In the same pan, add a bit more oil if needed.

  ii. Sauté garlic and ginger until fragrant.

  iii. Add mixed vegetables and stir-fry until they are tender-crisp.

6. Combine Tofu, Vegetables, and Quinoa:

  i. Add the cooked quinoa and sautéed tofu back to the pan with the vegetables.

7. Pour in Stir-Fry Sauce:

  i. Pour the prepared stir-fry sauce over the tofu, vegetables, and quinoa.

  ii. Toss everything together until well coated and heated through.

8. Finish and Garnish:

  i. Stir in sliced green onions.

  ii. Garnish with sesame seeds if desired.

9. Serve:

  i. Serve the Quinoa and Vegetable Stir-Fry with Tofu hot, and enjoy this wholesome and delicious plant-based meal.

10. Optional Additions:

  i. Add a sprinkle of red pepper flakes for some heat.

  ii. Include cashews or peanuts for extra crunch.

  iii. Garnish with cilantro or fresh lime wedges for added freshness.

Nutrition Information (Per Serving):

- Calories: 400

• Protein: 20g

• Carbohydrates: 45g

• Fat: 18g

• Saturated Fat: 2.5g

• Cholesterol: 0mg

• Fiber: 8g

• Sugar: 6g

• Sodium: 800mg

Whole Wheat Pasta with Tomato and Basil Sauce:

Meal Description: This Whole Wheat Pasta with Tomato and Basil Sauce is a classic and wholesome dish that combines the heartiness of whole wheat pasta with a flavorful homemade tomato and basil sauce. This meal is simple yet satisfying for a quick and nutritious weeknight dinner.

Ingredients:

For the Pasta:

• 8 ounces whole wheat pasta (spaghetti, penne, or your choice)

• Salt for boiling water

For the Tomato and Basil Sauce:

• Two tablespoons olive oil

• Three cloves garlic, minced

• One can (28 oz) crushed tomatoes

• One teaspoon dried oregano

• One teaspoon of dried basil

• Salt and pepper to taste

• Pinch of red pepper flakes (optional)

• Fresh basil leaves, chopped, for garnish

For Garnish:

• Grated Parmesan cheese (optional)

Instructions:

1. Cook Whole Wheat Pasta:
    i. Bring a large pot of salted water to a boil.
    ii. Cook the whole wheat pasta according to package instructions until al dente. Drain and set aside.
2. Prepare Tomato and Basil Sauce:
    i. In a large skillet, heat olive oil over medium heat.
    ii. Add minced garlic and sauté until fragrant but not browned.
3. Simmer Sauce:
    i. If using, pour in the crushed tomatoes, dried oregano, dried basil, salt, pepper, and red pepper flakes.
    ii. Stir to combine and bring the sauce to a simmer.
    iii. Let it simmer for 15-20 minutes to let the flavors meld and the sauce thicken slightly.
4. Toss Pasta in Sauce:
    i. Add the cooked whole wheat pasta to the skillet with the tomato and basil sauce.
    ii. Toss the pasta in the sauce until

well coated.

5. **Garnish and Serve:**
    i. Garnish the Whole Wheat Pasta with Tomato and Basil Sauce with chopped fresh basil.
    ii. Optionally, sprinkle with grated Parmesan cheese.

6. **Serve:**
    i. Serve the pasta hot, and enjoy the simplicity and richness of this delicious dish.

7. **Optional Additions:**
    i.   Add sautéed cherry tomatoes or sun-dried tomatoes for extra sweetness.
    ii. Include baby spinach or arugula for added greens.
    iii. Top with grilled chicken or shrimp for added protein.

Nutrition Information (Per Serving):

• Calories: 350

• Protein: 10g

• Carbohydrates: 60g

• Fat: 8g

• Saturated Fat: 1g

• Cholesterol: 0mg

• Fiber: 10g

• Sugar: 8g

• Sodium: 400mg

Brown Rice and Black Bean Burrito Bowl:

Meal Description: This Brown Rice and Black Bean Burrito Bowl is a nutritious and flavorful dish that combines wholesome brown rice, protein-packed black beans, and a variety of fresh toppings. Customize your bowl with colorful vegetables, creamy avocado, and zesty salsa for a delicious and satisfying meal.

Ingredients:

For the Brown Rice and Black Beans:

• 1 cup brown rice, cooked

• One can (15 oz) black beans, drained and rinsed

• One teaspoon of olive oil

• One teaspoon of ground cumin

• One teaspoon of chili powder

• Salt and pepper to taste

• Lime wedges for serving

For Toppings:

• Cherry tomatoes, halved

• Corn kernels, cooked

• Red onion, finely chopped

• Bell peppers, diced

• Avocado, sliced

• Fresh cilantro, chopped

• Salsa or pico de gallo

• Greek yogurt or sour cream (optional)

• Shredded cheese (cheddar or Mexican blend)

Instructions:

1. Cook Brown Rice:
    i. Cook brown rice according to package instructions.
2. Prepare Black Beans:
    i. In a skillet, heat olive oil over medium heat.
    ii. Add black beans, ground cumin, chili powder, salt, and pepper.
    iii. Cook for 5-7 minutes, stirring occasionally, until the beans are heated through and coated with the spices.
3. Assemble the Burrito Bowl:
    i. In serving bowls, layer cooked brown rice and seasoned black beans.
4. Add Toppings:
    i. Top with cherry tomatoes, corn kernels, red onion, diced bell peppers, sliced avocado, and fresh cilantro.
5. Squeeze Lime:
    i. Squeeze fresh lime wedges over the bowl for a burst of citrus flavor.
6. Drizzle with Salsa:
    i. Drizzle salsa or pico de gallo over the bowl for added zest.
7. Optional Garnishes:
    i. Add a dollop of Greek yogurt or sour cream if desired.
    ii. Sprinkle with shredded cheese for extra richness.

8. Mix and Enjoy:
    i. Gently mix the ingredients in the bowl to combine all the flavors.
    ii. Enjoy the Brown Rice and Black Bean Burrito Bowl immediately.
9. Optional Additions:
    i. Include grilled chicken, steak, or shrimp for added protein.
    ii. Toss in sautéed fajita vegetables for extra flavor.
    iii. Sprinkle with crushed tortilla chips for added crunch.

Nutrition Information (Per Serving):

- Calories: 400

- Protein: 12g

- Carbohydrates: 70g

- Fat: 8g

- Saturated Fat: 1g

- Cholesterol: 0mg

- Fiber: 12g

- Sugar: 3g

- Sodium: 500mg

Farro and Vegetable Pilaf with Grilled Chicken:

Meal Description: This Farro and Vegetable Pilaf with Grilled Chicken is a hearty and wholesome dish that combines nutty farro, a variety of colorful vegetables, and flavorful grilled chicken. Packed with protein, fiber, and a medley of textures, this pilaf makes for a satisfying and nutritious meal.

Ingredients:

For the Grilled Chicken:

• Two boneless, skinless chicken breasts

• Two tablespoons olive oil

• One teaspoon dried oregano

• One teaspoon of garlic powder

• Salt and pepper to taste

• Lemon wedges for serving

For the Farro and Vegetable Pilaf:

• 1 cup farro, rinsed

• 2 cups water or vegetable broth

• Two tablespoons olive oil

• One onion, finely chopped

• Two cloves garlic, minced

• One bell pepper, diced (any color)

• One zucchini, diced

• 1 cup cherry tomatoes, halved

• 1/2 cup frozen peas

• One teaspoon of dried thyme

• Salt and pepper to taste

• Fresh parsley, chopped, for garnish

Instructions:

1. Marinate and Grill Chicken:
   i. Combine olive oil, dried oregano, garlic powder, salt, and pepper in a bowl.

    ii. Coat the chicken breasts with the marinade and let them marinate for at least 30 minutes.

    iii. Grill the chicken breasts until fully cooked, about 6-8 minutes per side.

    iv. Slice the grilled chicken into strips and set aside.

2. Cook Farro:

    i. In a saucepan, combine farro and water or vegetable broth.

    ii. Bring to a boil, then reduce heat, cover, and simmer for 20-25 minutes or until the farro is tender but still has a chewy texture.

3. Sauté Vegetables:

    i. In a large skillet, heat olive oil over medium heat.

    ii. Add chopped onion and sauté until translucent.

    iii. Add minced garlic and sauté for an additional minute.

    iv. Add diced bell pepper, zucchini, cherry tomatoes, and frozen peas.

    v. Cook until the vegetables are tender but still vibrant.

4. Combine Farro and Vegetables:

    i. Add the cooked farro to the skillet with the sautéed vegetables.

    ii. Season with dried thyme, salt, and pepper.

    iii. Toss everything together until well combined.

5. Assemble Pilaf:
    i. Arrange the Farro and Vegetable Pilaf on serving plates.
    ii. Top with grilled chicken strips.
6. Garnish and Serve:
    i. Garnish with fresh chopped parsley.
    ii. Serve the pilaf hot, with lemon wedges on the side.
7. Optional Additions:
    i. Mix in crumbled feta or goat cheese for a creamy element.
    ii. Drizzle with balsamic glaze or a squeeze of lemon for added brightness.
    iii. Include a handful of toasted pine nuts or almonds for extra crunch.

Nutrition Information (Per Serving):

• Calories: 450

• Protein: 25g

• Carbohydrates: 50g

• Fat: 18g

• Saturated Fat: 3g

• Cholesterol: 50mg

• Fiber: 10g

• Sugar: 5g

• Sodium: 400mg

Oatmeal with Berries and Almonds:
Meal Description: This Oatmeal with Berries and Almonds

is a wholesome and nutritious breakfast option that combines the heartiness of oats with the sweetness of berries and the crunch of almonds. Packed with fiber, antioxidants, and healthy fats, this breakfast will keep you energized and satisfied throughout the morning.

Ingredients:

For the Oatmeal:

- 1 cup rolled oats

- 2 cups milk (dairy or plant-based)

- One tablespoon of honey or maple syrup (optional for sweetness)

- 1/2 teaspoon vanilla extract

- Pinch of salt

For Toppings:

- Mixed berries (strawberries, blueberries, raspberries)

- Sliced almonds

- Drizzle of honey or maple syrup

- Fresh mint leaves for garnish (optional)

Instructions:

Cook Oatmeal:

Combine rolled oats, milk, honey, or maple syrup (if using), vanilla extract, and a pinch of salt in a saucepan.

Bring the mixture to a simmer over medium heat.

Simmer Until Thickened:

Reduce the heat to low and simmer the

oatmeal, stirring occasionally, until it reaches your desired thickness.

Serve:

Divide the cooked oatmeal into serving bowls.

Add Toppings:

Top the oatmeal with a generous amount of mixed berries and sliced almonds.

Drizzle with Honey:

Drizzle honey or maple syrup over the berries and almonds for added sweetness.

Garnish and Enjoy:

Garnish with fresh mint leaves if desired.

Serve the Oatmeal with Berries and Almonds hot, and enjoy a nutritious and delicious breakfast.

Optional Variations:

For added richness, stir in a tablespoon of nut butter (almond butter, peanut butter).

Mix in chia seeds or flaxseeds and sprinkle for extra fiber and omega-3 fatty acids.

Include a dollop of Greek yogurt for added creaminess and protein.

Nutrition Information (Per Serving):

• Calories: 350

• Protein: 12g

• Carbohydrates: 55g

• Fat: 10g

• Saturated Fat: 2g

• Cholesterol: 10mg

• Fiber: 8g

• Sugar: 15g

• Sodium: 100mg

Whole Grain Wrap with Turkey and Hummus:

Meal Description: This Grain Wrap with Turkey and Hummus is a balanced and satisfying meal that combines lean turkey, creamy hummus, and a variety of fresh vegetables, all wrapped in a whole-grain tortilla. Packed with protein, fiber, and essential nutrients, this wrap is perfect for a quick and nutritious lunch or dinner.

Ingredients:

For the Wrap:

• One whole-grain tortilla or wrap

• 4 ounces lean turkey breast, thinly sliced

• Two tablespoons hummus (store-bought or homemade)

• 1/2 cup mixed salad greens (lettuce, spinach, arugula)

• 1/4 cup cherry tomatoes, halved

• 1/4 cucumber, thinly sliced

• Red onion, thinly sliced (optional)

• Sprouts or microgreens for garnish (optional)

Instructions:

1. Prepare the Ingredients:
    i. Lay out the whole-grain tortilla or wrap it on a clean surface.
2. Spread Hummus:
    i. Spread a generous layer of

hummus evenly over the entire surface of the tortilla.

3. Layer Turkey:

    i. Place the thinly sliced turkey breast over one-half of the tortilla.

4. Add Vegetables:

    i. Add mixed salad greens, cherry tomatoes, cucumber slices, and red onion (if using) over the turkey.

5. Fold and Roll:

    i. Starting from the side with the ingredients, fold in the sides of the tortilla, then roll it tightly from the bottom to create a wrap.

6. Slice and Garnish:

    i. If desired, slice the wrap in half diagonally for easier handling.

    ii. Garnish with sprouts or microgreens for an extra burst of freshness.

7. Serve:

    i. Serve the Whole Grain Wrap with Turkey and Hummus immediately, and enjoy a nutritious and flavorful meal.

8. Optional Variations:

    i. Add avocado slices for creaminess and healthy fats.

    ii. Drizzle with a balsamic glaze or your favorite dressing for extra flavor.

    iii. Include shredded carrots or bell peppers for added crunch.

Nutrition Information (Approximate):

• Calories: 350

• Protein: 25g

• Carbohydrates: 30g

• Fat: 15g

• Saturated Fat: 2.5g

• Cholesterol: 40mg

• Fiber: 6g

• Sugar: 3g

• Sodium: 600mg

Bulgur Salad with Chickpeas and Roasted Vegetables:

Meal Description: This Bulgur Salad with Chickpeas and Roasted Vegetables is a wholesome and flavorful dish that combines nutty Bulgur with protein-rich chickpeas and a medley of roasted vegetables. Tossed in a zesty vinaigrette, this salad is delicious and packed with essential nutrients.

Ingredients:

For the Salad:

• 1 cup coarse Bulgur

• 2 cups water or vegetable broth

• One can (15 oz) chickpeas, drained and rinsed

• One zucchini, diced

• One red bell pepper, diced

• One yellow bell pepper, diced

• One red onion, finely chopped

• Two tablespoons olive oil

- Salt and pepper to taste

For the Vinaigrette:

- Three tablespoons olive oil
- Two tablespoons of balsamic vinegar
- One teaspoon of Dijon mustard
- One clove of garlic, minced
- Salt and pepper to taste
- Fresh parsley, chopped, for garnish

Instructions:

1. Preheat Oven:
    i. Preheat the oven to 400°F (200°C).
2. Roast Vegetables:
    i. Toss diced zucchini, red bell pepper, yellow bell pepper, and finely chopped red onion with olive oil, salt, and pepper on a baking sheet.
    ii. Roast in the preheated oven for 20-25 minutes or until the vegetables are tender and slightly caramelized.
3. Cook Bulgur:
    i. In a saucepan, bring water or vegetable broth to a boil.
    ii. Add the bulge, reduce heat to low, cover it, and simmer it for 15-20 minutes or until it is cooked and has absorbed the liquid.
    iii. Fluff the cooked Bulgur with a fork.
4. Prepare Chickpeas:

      i. Combine drained and rinsed chickpeas in a bowl with a drizzle of olive oil, salt, and pepper.

5. Roast Chickpeas:
    i. Spread the seasoned chickpeas on a baking sheet and roast in the oven for 15-20 minutes or until they are crispy.

6. Make Vinaigrette:
    i. Whisk together olive oil, balsamic vinegar, Dijon mustard, minced garlic, salt, and pepper in a small bowl.

7. Assemble Salad:
    i. Combine the cooked Bulgur, roasted vegetables, and chickpeas in a large bowl.
    ii. Pour the vinaigrette over the salad and toss until everything is well coated.

8. Garnish and Serve:
    i. Garnish the Bulgur Salad with Chickpeas and Roasted Vegetables with chopped fresh parsley.
    ii. Serve the salad at room temperature or chilled.

9. Optional Additions:
    i. Toss in cherry tomatoes or sun-dried tomatoes for added sweetness.
    ii. Include crumbled feta or goat cheese for a creamy texture.
    iii. Top with toasted pine nuts or

almonds for extra crunch.

Nutrition Information (Approximate):

- Calories: 400
- Protein: 12g
- Carbohydrates: 60g
- Fat: 15g
- Saturated Fat: 2g
- Cholesterol: 0mg
- Fiber: 12g
- Sugar: 5g
- Sodium: 400mg

CHAPTER SEVEN

Hydration recipes

Infused Water with Cucumber and Mint:

Beverage Description: This Infused Water with Cucumber and Mint is a refreshing and hydrating drink that adds a burst of flavor to plain water. The crispness of cucumber combined with the refreshing aroma of mint creates a delightful and healthy beverage option.

Ingredients:

• 1/2 cucumber, thinly sliced

• Fresh mint leaves

• Ice cubes

• Water

Instructions:

1. Prepare Ingredients:
     i. Wash the cucumber thoroughly and slice it thinly.
     ii. Gather fresh mint leaves.
2. Assemble Infused Water:
     i. In a pitcher, combine the cucumber slices and fresh mint leaves.
3. Add Ice Cubes:
     i. Place ice cubes in the pitcher to keep the infused water cool.
4. Fill with Water:
     i. Fill the pitcher with water. Use filtered or cold water for the best taste.
5. Let it Infuse:
     i. Allow the water to infuse in the refrigerator for at least 1-2 hours.

> For a more intense flavor, you can leave it overnight.

6. Serve:

    i. Pour the infused water into glasses, ensuring some cucumber slices and mint leaves are in each serving.

7. Enjoy:

    i. Sip and enjoy this refreshing Infused Water with Cucumber and Mint as a hydrating and flavorful alternative to plain water.

Optional Variations:

• Add a squeeze of fresh lime or lemon for a citrusy twist.

• Include a few slices of ginger for a hint of warmth.

• Experiment with different herbs like basil or rosemary for unique flavors.

Benefits:

• Cucumber is hydrating and contains antioxidants.

• Mint is known for its refreshing properties and can aid in digestion.

Green Tea and Berry Smoothie:

Smoothie Description: This Green Tea and Berry Smoothie is a vibrant and antioxidant-rich blend that combines the goodness of green tea with the sweetness of mixed berries. This smoothie is a refreshing and healthy drink packed with vitamins and nutrients.

Ingredients:

• 1 cup brewed green tea, cooled

• 1/2 cup mixed berries (strawberries, blueberries,

raspberries)

- One banana, peeled and sliced

- 1 cup spinach leaves, washed

- 1/2 cup Greek yogurt (optional for creaminess)

- Honey or maple syrup to sweeten (optional)

- Ice cubes

Instructions:

1. Brew Green Tea:
   i. Brew a cup of green tea and allow it to cool. You can use bagged or loose-leaf green tea.
2. Prepare Ingredients:
   i. Wash the berries and spinach.
   ii. Peel and slice the banana.
3. Blend Ingredients:
   i. Combine the brewed and cooled green tea, mixed berries, sliced banana, spinach leaves, Greek yogurt (if using), and ice cubes in a blender.
4. Blend Until Smooth:
   i. Blend the ingredients until you achieve a smooth and creamy consistency.
5. Sweeten to Taste:
   i. Taste the smoothie and add honey or maple syrup if additional sweetness is desired. Blend again to combine.
6. Serve:
   i. Pour the Green Tea and Berry

Smoothie into glasses.

7. Garnish (Optional):

    i. Garnish with a few whole berries or a mint leaf for a decorative touch.

8. Enjoy:

    i. Sip and enjoy this refreshing and nutritious Green Tea and Berry Smoothie.

Optional Additions:

• Add a tablespoon of chia seeds or flaxseeds for extra fiber.

• Include a scoop of protein powder for added protein.

• Substitute coconut water for green tea for a different flavor profile.

Benefits:

• Green tea is rich in antioxidants and may offer various health benefits.

• Berries are high in vitamins, minerals, and antioxidants.

• Spinach provides a boost of vitamins and minerals.

Coconut Water and Pineapple Cooler:

Beverage Description: This Coconut Water and Pineapple Cooler is a tropical and hydrating drink that combines the natural sweetness of pineapple with the refreshing taste of coconut water. Packed with electrolytes and vitamins, this cooler is perfect for staying calm and refreshed.

Ingredients:

• 1 cup fresh pineapple chunks

• 1 cup coconut water

• Ice cubes

• Mint leaves for garnish (optional)

• Pineapple slices for garnish (optional)

Instructions:

1. Prepare Ingredients:
    i. Peel and cut fresh pineapple into chunks.
2. Blend Pineapple:
    i. In a blender, add the fresh pineapple chunks.
3. Add Coconut Water:
    i. Pour coconut water over the pineapple in the blender.
4. Blend Until Smooth:
    i. Blend the pineapple and coconut water until you achieve a smooth consistency.
5. Strain (Optional):
    i. If desired, strain the mixture to remove the pulp for a smoother texture.
6. Serve Over Ice:
    i. Fill glasses with ice cubes.
7. Pour the Cooler:
    i. Pour the blended pineapple and coconut water mixture over the ice.
8. Garnish (Optional):
    i. Garnish the Coconut Water and Pineapple Cooler with mint leaves or pineapple slices for an extra touch of freshness.
9. Stir (Optional):

                          i. Give it a gentle stir with a spoon to mix the flavors.

10. Enjoy:

                          i. Sip and enjoy this tropical and hydrating Coconut Water and Pineapple Cooler.

Optional Additions:

• Add a splash of lime juice for a citrusy kick.

• Include a pinch of salt for an electrolyte boost.

• Blend in a few mint leaves for added flavor.

Benefits:

• Coconut water is hydrating and rich in electrolytes.

• Pineapple provides natural sweetness and is a good source of vitamin C.

Watermelon Mint Lemonade:

Beverage Description: This Watermelon Mint Lemonade is a refreshing and hydrating drink that combines the juicy sweetness of watermelon with the zesty tang of lemons, all infused with the cooling essence of fresh mint. Perfect for hot days or as a delightful party beverage.

Ingredients:

• 4 cups fresh watermelon, cubed and seedless

• 1 cup freshly squeezed lemon juice (about 4-6 lemons)

• 1/2 cup fresh mint leaves, loosely packed

• 1/4 cup honey or agave syrup (adjust to taste)

• 4 cups cold water

• Ice cubes

• Lemon slices and mint sprigs for garnish

Instructions:

1. Prepare Ingredients:
    i. Cube the watermelon, ensuring it's seedless.
    ii. Squeeze lemons to obtain fresh lemon juice.
2. Blend Watermelon:
    i. In a blender, puree the fresh watermelon until smooth.
3. Strain (Optional):
    i. You can strain the watermelon puree to remove pulp if you prefer a smoother texture.
4. Muddle Mint Leaves:
    i. In a pitcher, muddle the fresh mint leaves to release their flavor.
5. Mix Ingredients:
    i. Add the strained watermelon puree, freshly squeezed lemon juice, honey or agave syrup, and cold water to the pitcher.
6. Stir Well:
    i. Stir the mixture well to combine all the ingredients.
7. Taste and Adjust:
    i. Taste the Watermelon Mint Lemonade and adjust sweetness by adding more honey or agave syrup if needed.
8. Chill:
    i. Refrigerate the lemonade for at least 1-2 hours to allow the flavors to meld.

9. Serve Over Ice:

> i. Fill glasses with ice cubes.

10. Pour and Garnish:

> i. Pour the chilled Watermelon Mint Lemonade over the ice.
>
> ii. Garnish each glass with a slice of lemon and a sprig of mint.

11. Stir Before Serving (Optional):

> i. Give the lemonade a gentle stir before serving to distribute the mint flavor.

12. Enjoy:

> i. Sip and enjoy this cool and revitalizing Watermelon Mint Lemonade.

Optional Additions:

• Add a splash of sparkling water for a fizzy version.

• Include a few cucumber slices for an extra refreshing twist.

Benefits:

• Watermelon is hydrating and contains vitamins A and C.

• Lemon provides a dose of vitamin C and adds a tangy flavor.

• Mint contributes a refreshing and cooling element.

Herbal Iced Tea with Citrus:

Beverage Description: This Herbal Iced Tea with Citrus is a refreshing and caffeine-free drink that combines a blend of herbal teas with the citrusy zing of oranges and lemons. Perfect for a sunny day or as a hydrating option at gatherings.

Ingredients:

• Four herbal tea bags (such as peppermint, chamomile, or hibiscus)

• One orange, thinly sliced

• One lemon, thinly sliced

• 1/4 cup honey or agave syrup (adjust to taste)

• Fresh mint leaves for garnish (optional)

• Ice cubes

• 4 cups boiling water

Instructions:

1. Boil Water:
    i. Bring 4 cups of water to a boil.
2. Brew Herbal Tea:
    i. Place the herbal tea bags in a heatproof pitcher.
    ii. Pour the boiling water over the tea bags.
    iii. Let the tea steep for 5-7 minutes or according to the package instructions.
3. Add Citrus Slices:
    i. While the tea is still warm, add thinly sliced oranges and lemons to the pitcher.
4. Sweeten the Tea:
    i. Stir in honey or agave syrup to sweeten the tea. Adjust the sweetness to your liking.
5. Cool and Chill:
    i. Allow the tea to cool to room

temperature, then refrigerate until well chilled.

6. Serve Over Ice:
    i. Fill glasses with ice cubes.
7. Pour and Garnish:
    i. Pour the chilled Herbal Iced Tea with Citrus over the ice.
    ii. Garnish each glass with a slice of orange or lemon and fresh mint leaves if desired.
8. Stir Before Serving (Optional):
    i. Give the iced tea a gentle stir before serving to distribute the citrus flavors.
9. Enjoy:
    i. Sip and enjoy this delightful Herbal Iced Tea with Citrus as an excellent and revitalizing beverage.

Optional Additions:

• Include a splash of ginger syrup for a hint of warmth.

• Add a few slices of cucumber for an extra refreshing element.

Benefits:

• Herbal teas may offer various health benefits depending on the herbs used.

• Citrus fruits provide a boost of vitamin C and add a bright, citrusy flavor.

Strawberry Basil Sparkling Water:

Beverage Description: This Strawberry Basil Sparkling Water is a refreshing and vibrant drink that combines the sweetness of ripe strawberries with the herbal notes of fresh basil, all topped off with effervescent sparkling water. Perfect for a light and flavorful hydration option.

Ingredients:

• 1 cup fresh strawberries, hulled and halved

• 1/4 cup fresh basil leaves, torn

• One tablespoon of honey or agave syrup (optional for sweetness)

• Sparkling water

• Ice cubes

• Strawberry slices and basil sprigs for garnish (optional)

Instructions:

1. Prepare Ingredients:
    i. Hull and halve fresh strawberries.
    ii. Tear fresh basil leaves.
2. Muddle Strawberries and Basil:
    i. Muddle the fresh strawberries and torn basil leaves together in a glass or pitcher to release their flavors.
3. Sweeten (Optional):
    i. Add honey or agave syrup to sweeten the strawberry and basil mixture if desired. Stir to combine.
4. Add Ice Cubes:
    i. Fill the glass or pitcher with ice cubes.
5. Pour Sparkling Water:
    i. Pour sparkling water over the muddled strawberries, basil, and ice.
6. Stir Gently:

    i. Give the mixture a gentle stir to distribute the flavors.

7. Garnish (Optional):
    i. Garnish the Strawberry Basil Sparkling Water with slices of fresh strawberries and sprigs of basil.

8. Serve Immediately:
    i. Serve the sparkling water immediately while it's effervescent and refreshing.

9. Enjoy:
    i. Sip and enjoy this delightful Strawberry Basil Sparkling Water as a fruity and herbal beverage.

Optional Additions:

• Add a freshly squeezed lime or lemon juice splash for extra citrusy brightness.

• Include a few slices of cucumber for a relaxed and crisp twist.

Benefits:

• Strawberries are rich in vitamin C and antioxidants.

• Basil adds a unique herbal flavor and may have potential health benefits.

Ginger Lemon Turmeric Infusion:

Beverage Description: This Ginger Lemon Turmeric Infusion is a warming and immune-boosting drink that combines the anti-inflammatory properties of turmeric with the zesty kick of fresh lemon and the spicy warmth of ginger. This infusion is not only delicious but also offers potential health benefits.

Ingredients:

• 1-inch piece of fresh ginger, thinly sliced

• One teaspoon ground turmeric or 1-inch piece of fresh turmeric, thinly sliced

• One lemon, thinly sliced

• One tablespoon of honey or agave syrup (adjust to taste)

• 4 cups hot water

Instructions:

1. Prepare Ingredients:
    i. Thinly slice the fresh ginger, turmeric, and lemon.
2. Combine in a Teapot or Pitcher:
    i. Place the sliced ginger, turmeric, and lemon in a teapot or heatproof pitcher.
3. Add Hot Water:
    i. Pour hot water over the ginger, turmeric, and lemon slices.
4. Steep:
    i. Allow the infusion to steep for 10-15 minutes to extract the flavors and beneficial compounds.
5. Sweeten (Optional):
    i. Add honey or agave syrup to sweeten the infusion. Stir well to dissolve.
6. Strain (Optional):
    i. Strain the infusion to remove the ginger, turmeric, and lemon pieces if desired.
7. Serve:

        i. Pour the Ginger Lemon Turmeric Infusion into cups.

8. Garnish (Optional):
   i. Garnish each cup with a slice of lemon or a sprinkle of turmeric for a decorative touch.
9. Sip and Enjoy:
   i. Sip on this warming and immune-boosting infusion to enjoy its delightful flavors and potential health benefits.

Optional Additions:

• Include a pinch of black pepper, which may enhance the absorption of turmeric's active compound, curcumin.

• Add a cinnamon stick for an extra layer of warmth and flavor.

Benefits:

• Ginger has anti-inflammatory and antioxidant properties.

• Turmeric contains curcumin, which is known for its potential health benefits.

• Lemon provides vitamin C and adds a refreshing citrusy flavor.

Berry and Mint Detox Water:

Beverage Description: This Berry and Mint Detox Water is a refreshing and hydrating drink that combines the natural sweetness of berries with the vital essence of fresh mint. Packed with antioxidants and vitamins, this detox water is a delightful way to stay hydrated.

Ingredients:

• 1 cup mixed berries (strawberries, blueberries,

raspberries)

- 1/4 cup fresh mint leaves

- Ice cubes

- Water

Instructions:

1. Prepare Ingredients:
     i. Wash the berries and mint leaves.
2. Muddle Berries and Mint:
     i. Muddle the mixed berries and fresh mint leaves in a pitcher to release their flavors.
3. Add Ice Cubes:
     i. Fill the pitcher with ice cubes.
4. Fill with Water:
     i. Pour water over the muddled berries, mint, and ice.
5. Stir Gently:
     i. Give the mixture a gentle stir to combine the ingredients.
6. Chill:
     i. Refrigerate the Berry and Mint Detox Water for at least 1-2 hours to allow the flavors to infuse.
7. Serve Over Ice:
     i. Fill glasses with ice cubes.
8. Pour and Garnish:
     i. Pour the chilled detox water over the ice.
     ii. Garnish each glass with a few whole berries and mint leaves if desired.

9. Stir Before Serving (Optional):

    i. Give the detox water a gentle stir before serving to distribute the flavors.

10. Sip and Enjoy:

    i. Sip on this refreshing Berry and Mint Detox Water as a hydrating and antioxidant-rich beverage.

Optional Additions:

• Add a few slices of cucumber for extra freshness.

• Include a splash of lime or lemon juice for a citrusy kick.

Benefits:

• Berries are rich in antioxidants and vitamins.

• Mint is known for its digestive properties and adds a refreshing flavor.

CONCLUSION

In conclusion, the mesothelioma diet represents a crucial aspect of the comprehensive care and support required by individuals facing the challenges of this aggressive cancer. While no single dietary regimen can eradicate mesothelioma, the role of nutrition in mitigating symptoms, supporting overall health, and improving the quality of life during treatment is undeniable. This exploration into the mesothelioma diet has underscored the importance of a personalized and holistic approach, considering individual health conditions, treatment plans, and nutritional needs.

The journey through mesothelioma is arduous, marked by medical complexities and emotional strains. The mesothelioma diet serves as a tool for empowerment, allowing individuals to actively participate in their well-being by making informed dietary choices. By addressing nutritional requirements, managing treatment-related side effects, and supporting the body's resilience, a thoughtfully designed diet can contribute to a more positive and robust response to the challenges posed by mesothelioma.

www.ingramcontent.com/pod-product-compliance
Lightning Source LLC
Chambersburg PA
CBHW050729260726
48661CB00001B/138